UNDOCUMENTED MIGRANTS AND HEALTHCARE

Undocumented Migrants and Healthcare

Eight Stories from Switzerland

Marianne Jossen

OpenBook Publishers

https://www.openbookpublishers.com

© 2018 Marianne Jossen

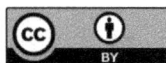

Open Reports Series, vol. 6 | ISSN: 2399-6668 (Print); 2399-6676 (Online)

ISBN Paperback: 978-1-78374-478-7
ISBN Hardback: 978-1-78374-479-4
ISBN Digital (PDF): 978-1-78374-480-0
ISBN Digital ebook (epub): 978-1-78374-481-7
ISBN Digital ebook (mobi): 978-1-78374-482-4
DOI: 10.11647/OBP.0139

The Stiftung Lindenhof Bern and the Swiss Red Cross have generously contributed to this publication.

Cover image: *Ambulance Pan* (2010). Photo by Justin S. Campbell, CC BY-ND 2.0, https://www.flickr.com/photos/29143375@N05/5031411969. Cover design: Anna Gatti

All paper used by Open Book Publishers is SFI (Sustainable Forestry Initiative), PEFC (Programme for the Endorsement of Forest Certification Schemes) and Forest Stewardship Council(r)(FSC(r) certified.

Printed in the United Kingdom, United States, and Australia
by Lightning Source for Open Book Publishers (Cambridge, UK)

Contents

Acknowledgments

I would like to thank Kristen Jafflin, Sajida Ally, Jessica Potter, Thomas Abel and my peer reviewers for their inspiring comments. Thanks to Cindy-Jane Armbruster, Clara Benn, Alex Colville and Lucy Barnes for proof-reading the manuscript. Thanks also to Open Book Publishers for the professional handling of the publication. And thanks to my friends and family, and especially to Lukas, for listening to my stories over and over again.

Last but not least, thanks go to the medical and administrative professionals at the NGOs, and others based elsewhere, who gave their time for interviews. My greatest thanks, however, go to the undocumented migrants for agreeing to share their stories and a part of their lives with me.

1. Just going to hospital

January 2016. It is about two months since I wrote an introductory email to Julia,[1] the head of a department of an NGO that caters to the healthcare needs of so-called undocumented migrants in a Swiss region. In my email, I asked whether I might be able to undertake some volunteering and research. Since meeting Julia, I have done some translation work for the NGO, and now she has told me that if I am interested I can accompany some undocumented migrants on their hospital visits.

This is the first time Julia has asked me to perform such a task. The patient, Nicolas, needs an examination at a public hospital in the area. On the phone Julia reassures me that everything should go smoothly, as Nicolas has insurance. He will bring the contract to prove it, but he has no insurance card. All in all, she tells me, it would be good to have somebody with Nicolas who 'can explain things in a good, broad Swiss accent' (as Julia puts it).

She had instructed Nicolas to meet me in front of the hospital one and a half hours before the appointment–he has never been to this hospital before and therefore needs to be registered first. 'It's better to be early, just in case…' advises Julia. She reminds me to call her if there are any problems.

One morning three days later I meet Nicolas in front of the hospital. He hands me all the paperwork he has brought along. I find a referral letter, an insurance contract, and some medical results that I avoid looking at. I feel like an intruder into a stranger's privacy. We walk to

---

1   Everyone mentioned in this report has been given a pseudonym. See Chapter Three for further information.

     https://doi.org/10.11647/OBP.0139.01

the reception, where I show the papers. We are sent to another desk for registration.

On arrival I explain that I am here to accompany this patient. I address the receptionist in one of the Swiss national languages while Nicolas uses another one. The receptionist asks me for the insurance card. I reply that Nicolas does not have one, but that he has brought along his policy documents. 'Normally we need that card', she says. I do not respond. Then the receptionist asks for the patient's address. I tell her that she can use the address on the policy, but she points out that it includes only a post-box address. She insists that surely the man must be living somewhere. I agree and then reiterate that this is the only address available. I am suddenly uncertain. Would Nicolas really be risking anything by giving the hospital his address? I am not sure. Finally the receptionist says, quite sharply: 'So, he lives nowhere'. 'Exactly', I respond drily.

We continue. An emergency contact is listed on the insurance policy. Still, the employee needs a phone number. Nicolas provides one. The receptionist does not understand it, so I translate. A few sentences later, as I continue to translate Nicolas' explanations, she interrupts me, telling me that she understands Nicolas just fine.

Finally, she asks for an identity card. I explain that he does not have one. She tells me that she has to clarify this with her manager. I am worried about the tense atmosphere that has developed between us, so I tell her I understand and that she can call the NGO for further information.

On her return, the receptionist says that her manager has given his approval, but she needs to know whether Nicolas is a failed asylum seeker or if he is still going through the asylum process. I say that his status has not yet been determined. She accepts this and we are free to leave.

I accompany Nicolas over to the waiting area. A doctor arrives to call him in, at which point we say goodbye.

Outside, I feel relieved and upset at the same time. I ask myself a number of questions: How does Nicolas feel, having to hand over his personal documents to a complete stranger, then letting that stranger take the lead in such a supposedly easy task as hospital registration? Why does he have no insurance card even though he has insurance?

How did he obtain this insurance and how does he pay for it? Does he face similar difficulties when trying to register for other healthcare services? Is he eligible for state subsidies for his insurance, like low-income Swiss citizens? Why is the NGO listed as his correspondence address? Why did the receptionist react so emotionally to the missing insurance card and residential address, and why were my responses similarly emotional? I wonder about how his appointment with the doctor might be going. Then, my questions begin to broaden in scope. Do other undocumented migrants face similar situations? Might some of them not even have insurance? What happens then? If they do not know about the NGO, do they go to the emergency department?

This book aims to answer these questions. After outlining the situation of undocumented migrants and their access to healthcare in Europe (and particularly in Switzerland) in Chapter Two, I shall explain my research methodology and theoretical perspective in Chapter Three, while also introducing the NGO and its work. In Chapters Four to Six, the reader will embark on a journey through the worlds of eight undocumented migrants who have shared their experiences of healthcare in Switzerland. Their stories have been collected at and around the NGO, and they are augmented by the words of healthcare professionals.

2. Undocumented migrants, healthcare and health

In this chapter, I shall provide some contextual information about undocumented migrants in Europe. I discuss concepts of 'undocumentedness', and various estimates of the number of undocumented people, as well as outlining healthcare policies and practices across a number of European countries, with a particular focus on Switzerland. I will also address the question of undocumented migrants' health issues.

Estimates of the uncountable and concepts of the unnamed

Lacking the legal entitlement to stay in a country, undocumented migrants have been described as 'formally excluded, but physically present within the state's territory' (Karlsen 2016:136). The category generally includes those who have overstayed their visas, people who crossed the border without legal entitlement to do so, and failed asylum seekers (Kotsioni 2016).

Undocumented migrants' names therefore do not appear in official state registers, as their movements across countries are rarely tracked by the authorities and no census reaches them. Furthermore, and as we will see in greater detail below, the multiple and ever-changing categories describing a person's legal status make it difficult to produce accurate data (see Jandl 2004 for further details). Because of these difficulties,

 https://doi.org/10.11647/OBP.0139.02

research can produce only rough estimates about the number of undocumented migrants. The International Organization for Migration (IOM) estimates that in 2010, worldwide, about 10–15% of the estimated 214 million international migrants went undocumented (IOM 2010). The Clandestino Project estimated that in 2008, between 1.9 and 3.8 million undocumented migrants lived in the European Union (at that time comprising twenty-seven countries). This equates to approximately 0.39–0.77% of the total population and 7–13% of the foreign population (Clandestino Project 2009; Vogel et al. 2011). The Clandestino Project provides the highest and lowest estimates for a number of countries, as Figure 1 shows.

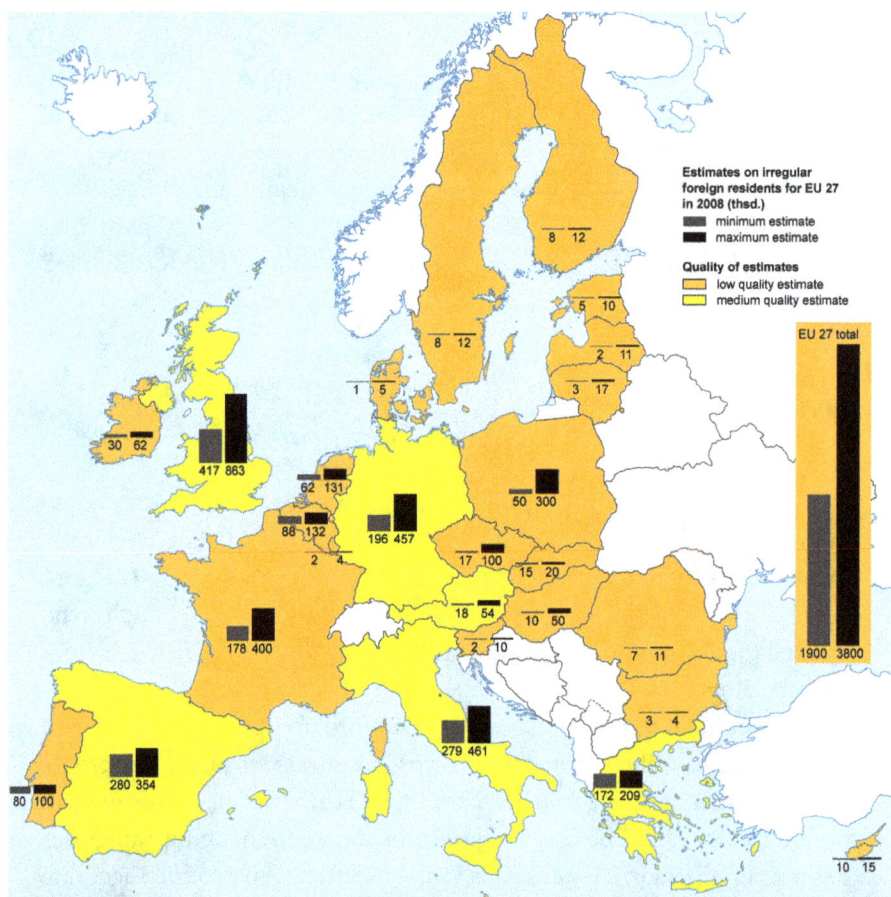

Fig. 1 Estimates of undocumented migrants in 2008. Graphic by Marcel Waldvogel based on data from the Clandestino Project (2009) and on a map by Wikimedia-Commons-User Alexrk2, https://commons.wikimedia.org/wiki/File:Europe_blank_laea_location_map.svg

Some updated numbers have become available in the interim (Clandestino Project 2017), pointing to a rise in numbers, as the table below shows.

Country	Estimates in 2008	Updated estimates (year of update)
Germany	178,000–400,000	180,000–520,000 (2015)
Greece	172,000–209,000	390,000 (2011)
Spain	280,000–354,000	300,000–390,000 (2009)

Fig. 2 Latest updates concerning the number of undocumented migrants with comparison to estimates of 2008, according to the Clandestino Project (2017).

Accordingly, the Frontex Annual Risk Analyses show increases in most of the indicators of irregular migration flows in the EU from both 2013–2014 and 2014–2015 (Frontex 2015; 2016). The table below shows examples of two of these indicators: refusal of entry to the EU and detected illegal border crossings.

Indicator	2014	2015
Refusal of entry to the EU	144,887	188,495
Detected illegal border crossings	282,962	1,822,337

Fig. 3 Indicators for irregular migration in 2014 and 2015, according to Frontex (2016).

However, the category of illegal border crossings includes not only those who go undocumented, but everyone who asks for asylum. Moreover there were more people who crossed the border and subsequently asked for asylum in 2015 than in the year before. It is therefore difficult to determine the exact increase in undocumented migrants.

The most recent estimates for Switzerland can be found in a state-commissioned study by Morlok et al. (2015). While an earlier study, also commissioned by the government, estimated a population of 90,000 undocumented migrants in 2005 (Longchamp 2005), Morlok et al. (2015) give a lower estimate of 76,000 undocumented migrants for 2015, a figure based on various sources of information. As Figure 4 shows, the estimate is extrapolated from expert interviews. The experts estimated the number of undocumented migrants to range between 58,000 and 105,000. The number is further contextualised using analyses of the number of known fatalities and births of persons without residency in Switzerland.

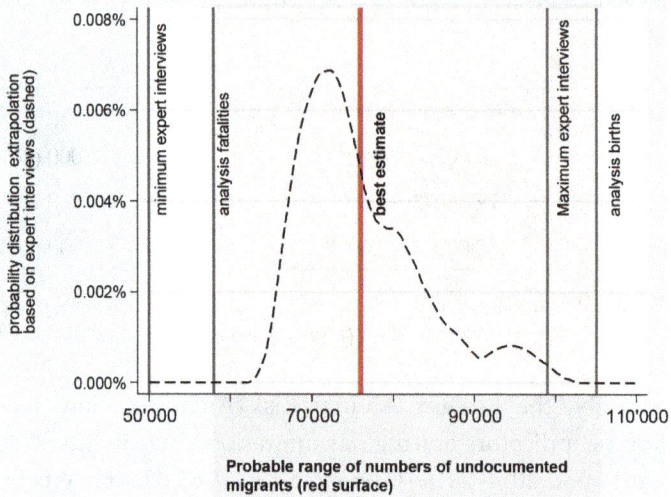

Fig. 4 Estimates of undocumented migrants in Switzerland in 2014.
Graphic reproduced with permission from Morlok et al. (2015).

Morlok et al. (2015) further estimated that two thirds (63%) of the undocumented migrants entered the country without permission to do so, or overstayed their tourist visa. The final third is made up of individuals who lost their legal right to stay after longer periods of time, for example after a divorce (18%), as well as failed asylum seekers (19%). It is further estimated that about 43% of undocumented migrants in Switzerland were born in South America, while 24% originated in Europe, with a further 19% coming from Africa and 11% from Asia. The majority are between eighteen and forty years old. About 41% have received only a basic education, between six and nine years of primary school. The remaining 59% have received secondary education–a three to four-year apprenticeship–or higher education such as a university degree.

This said, it is important to keep in mind that being undocumented is not a personal characteristic but a social construct. In the words of Bloch et al. undocumented migration results from

the interplay between restructured labour markets and increasingly complex migration controls and categories [that] created the interstices within which undocumented migrants found space. (2014:17)

This point can be illustrated with a closer look at Swiss immigration policy. In twentieth-century Switzerland, it is significant that immigration has been framed mostly as a labour issue. For instance, until 2002, the country ran a seasonal workers scheme that allowed foreigners to work in Switzerland for a nine-month period before having to return to their countries of origin for at least four months. Switching places of employment during this nine-month period was forbidden and seasonal workers, also known as *saisonniers*, had limited access to social security. Only after having worked in Switzerland for four consecutive seasons could a *saisonnier* obtain a residential permit (Arlettaz 2017). This state of affairs was criticized as inhumane from its inception (Piguet 2013:39). When the scheme was abandoned in 2002 with the introduction of free movement for European citizens, an unknown number of former seasonal workers stayed on and became undocumented migrants. The example of these former *saisonniers* clearly demonstrates that the status of being an undocumented migrant is a legal construct, and the laws that shape this status can change over time (see also Zimmermann 2011; Castaneda et al. 2015; Karlsen 2016).

It is important to note that being undocumented is a process (see Bloch et al. 2014). This means firstly that a person's status can shift from legal to undocumented and back again, with accompanying grey areas and transition periods. As a consequence, estimates about the number of undocumented migrants at any given time must always be taken with a pinch of salt.

Secondly, to view someone as undocumented means focusing not only on their legal status but also its effects upon their daily life. Being undocumented is thus never a full description of a person, but rather a social construct.

In this study, the concept of being 'undocumented' refers to how people deal with this social construct. The retelling of the undocumented migrants' stories will both rely on and illuminate the dynamic nature of the migrants' legal status.

Healthcare for undocumented migrants: policies…

Having introduced definitions and estimates, as well as having explored the shifting state of being undocumented, we will turn to the macro-social forces, namely the policies, that define and shape healthcare for undocumented migrants. As we will see, these policies vary in several ways. This section will give a sense of how such variety comes about–the result of principles and mechanisms that differ in content, time and space. This discussion will help contextualise the example of Switzerland, which is explored at the end of this section, demonstrating that it is important to discuss policies in relation to local situations.

Healthcare systems are often classified by how they are financed. In Europe, there are two main systems: the Bismarck system, which sets up healthcare via health insurance plans, and the Beveridge system, which is a tax-funded national health service.

How does this affect healthcare policies for undocumented migrants? Fundamentally, tax-based systems ensure that eligibility for care is based on residency. Beyond this, the circumstances in which non-residents are eligible for care must be defined. Within insurance-based systems, the question arises as to who is entitled and/or obliged to take out insurance, and what kind of care those who have not taken out insurance (a category that often includes undocumented migrants) should be afforded.

Björngren Cuadra & Cattacin (2011) classify European countries that follow the Beveridge and Bismarck systems according to the degree of access to healthcare they grant to undocumented migrants. In their classification, a 'no rights' policy makes accessing even emergency healthcare impossible. They would also describe as 'no rights' policies those in which the attempt to acquire insurance would burden a person with prohibitive debt. A 'minimum rights' policy grants access to emergency care. Finally, a 'more than minimum rights' approach allows access to both primary and secondary care.

The Platform for International Cooperation on Undocumented Migrants (PICUM) gives details about the policies that regulate undocumented migrants' access to healthcare in eleven European countries (PICUM 2007). The authors divide countries into five categories (Figure 5 below), ranging from those where 'all care is provided only on a payment basis' (category i), to those toying with the idea of 'free access to healthcare for all, including undocumented migrants' (category v). Between the two extremes lie countries proposing free access only in limited cases (category ii), and countries offering somewhat broader coverage (category iii). Furthermore, some countries (category iv), have set up a parallel administrative and payment system specifically for undocumented migrants (PICUM 2007:8).

System	Country	Classification PICUM (2007)	Classification Björngren Cuadra & Cattacin (2011)
Tax	Sweden	category i	
	Finland		No rights
	Ireland		
	Malta		
Insurance	Bulgaria		
	Czech Republic		
	Latvia		No rights
	Luxembourg		
	Romania		
Tax	Cyprus		
	Denmark		Minimum rights
	UK	category iii	
Insurance	Lithuania		
	Austria	category i	
	Belgium	category iv	
	Estonia		
	Germany	category ii	
	Greece		Minimum rights
	Hungary	category ii	
	Poland		
	Slovak Republic		
	Slovenia		
Tax	Italy	category v	
	Spain	category v	Rights
	Portugal	category iii	
Insurance	France	category iv	
	Netherlands	category iv	Rights
	Switzerland		

Fig. 5 Classification of policies concerning healthcare for undocumented migrants, according to PICUM (2007) and Björngren Cuadra & Cattacin (2011).

As this table shows, there appear to be differences between these two systems of classification; however, these can be explained after a closer look. For example, Austria is placed in the lowest category by PICUM, whereas according to Björngren-Cuadra & Cattacin, they would at least grant emergency care to undocumented migrants. Still, in their more detailed analysis, the latter argue that the situation could also be classified as 'no rights' because patients run the risk of accumulating a high debt when seeking healthcare. In the case of Switzerland, the authors mention that the high insurance fees present a significant obstacle for this segment of the population when trying to access healthcare provision.

The classifications provide an insight into the intricate policies that govern healthcare for undocumented migrants and invite us to have a closer look at the variations between them.

To start with, it is important to note that not all countries have specific policies to deal with this issue, despite their having ratified international human rights laws (Biswas et al. 2012). For example, in Denmark 'policies and legislation on undocumented migrants' medical rights appear ambiguous and are only sporadically described by decision-making bodies' (Biswas et al. 2011). It is unclear to what extent healthcare in Denmark must be provided beyond emergency services and whether or not undocumented migrants can be charged for it.

Insofar as policies are formulated, they sometimes only take specific groups of undocumented migrants into account. Thus, in Sweden until 2013, adult undocumented migrants were charged even for emergency healthcare (Verein SansPapiersCare 2016). Meanwhile, children who had not been granted asylum could nonetheless obtain some financial aid (Björngren-Cuadra 2012:115). In Norway, healthcare provision is restricted to emergency-only care for undocumented migrants as well as for short-term working immigrants (Ruud et al. 2015).

In other countries, access is granted to all types of undocumented migrants, but only for specific concerns and/or for a certain period of time. In the UK, undocumented migrants have access to primary and emergency care without charge (Sigona & Hughes 2012:11), while secondary care, involving treatment by specialists or in a hospital, is only delivered upon payment. The Migrant and Visitor Cost Recovery Programme implemented by the UK Government takes further steps to ensure that migrants pay for their own healthcare (Britz & McKee 2015). In Germany, undocumented migrants have access to healthcare during the first forty-eight months of their stay 'in cases of serious illness or acute pain' (Björngren-Cuadra 2012:118). Additionally, they have access to perinatal care, vaccinations, and sexual health screenings and care.

Policies and studies on the health and healthcare of undocumented migrants often focus on communicable diseases and reproductive health, which reflects the traditional importance of this area of public health, but which has nonetheless attracted criticism (Bivins 2015). This trend can also be observed in Italy, where from 1996 to 2001 the law gave migrants access to 'specific services such as pregnancy care, the protection of minors, prophylaxis, and vaccinations' (Piccoli 2016:15), whilst otherwise remaining ambiguous about the level of healthcare to which they were entitled.

The example of Italy also reveals other elements that have to be taken into account when conducting policy studies: namely changes to policies over time, together with regional differences. Indeed, in 2001, a constitutional reform gave Italian regions exclusive discretion over healthcare. This resulted in a highly fragmented landscape, in which twelve regional governments introduced varying policies ranging from 'strong activism' in Tuscany to 'relative inaction' in Lombardy (Piccoli 2016:15).

Similarly, in Sweden, a law introduced in 2013 allows treatment of urgent health problems for a nominal fee of five euros. Since then, regional district councils have also been able to grant undocumented migrants the same access to healthcare as citizens (Verein SansPapiersCare 2016). The question of access is thus, once again, regionalized.

Spain provides another very good example of these transformations: in 2012, a widely criticized (Casino 2012; Legido-Quigley 2013) Royal Decree Law revoked the previous right to full healthcare for undocumented migrants, limiting it to some exceptions. Many of the autonomous regions, however

> adopted legal, legislative and administrative actions to void or limit [the law's] effects, while others applied it as intended, resulting in huge differences in healthcare coverage for irregular migrants among Spanish Regions. (Cimas et al. 2016)

In Switzerland, healthcare is generally regulated by the national law on health insurance, the 'Krankenversicherungsgesetz' (KVG). Switzerland has a strong federal tradition, so its administrative regions, the cantons, retain much of the power to implement this law and regulate healthcare autonomously in their areas. Furthermore, private companies are heavily involved — generalists' and specialists' practices are privately owned and increasing numbers of hospitals also tend to be privatized. The system is thus influenced by both public and private interests (see also Rossini & Legrand-Germanier 2010; De Pietro et al. 2015; Marks-Sultan et al. 2016).

Healthcare is organized via an insurance scheme, participation in which is obligatory for everyone who resides in the country for more than three months. The insurance is provided by private companies, which are legally obliged to use the profits only for the provision of healthcare services to their insured clients. A basic insurance scheme covers primary and secondary care, pre- and post-natal care, reproductive care, psychotherapy — if prescribed by a general practitioner–preventative healthcare and rehabilitation. Dental care is not covered.

Premiums for these basic insurance schemes differ regionally and depend on the individual insurance policy. Policies that limit the patient's choice of doctors, for example, are available at reduced prices. Additionally, the insured person has to choose an annual excess ranging from 300 to 2,500 Swiss francs (CHF). A higher excess results in a cheaper premium. On top of this excess the patient must pay out of pocket for 10% of their treatment up to a maximum of CHF 700. Those in reduced financial circumstances can apply for premium subsidies from the state, the amount of which again varies depending on the region (see Chapter Four for a specific example). Those without insurance are still entitled to 'assistance when in need' (*Federal Constitution of the Swiss Confederation*, Art. 12). Whether this encompasses more than aid in life-threatening situations is subject to debate (Bilger et al. 2011).

According to current policy interpretations, undocumented migrants in Switzerland have both the right and the duty to take out insurance, because they reside in the country (*Swiss Civil Code*, Art. 23–26; *Verordnung über die Krankenversicherung*, Art. 1 al. 1; *Bundesgesetz über den Allgemeinen Teil des Sozialversicherungsrechts*, Art. 13). In 2002, the Federal Social Insurance Office issued an order that threatened sanctions against insurance companies that refused to accept undocumented migrants (Federal Social Insurance Office 2002). These included fines of up to CHF 5,000 and the possibility of legal action in cases of violation of professional discretion. But for undocumented migrants, as for all those who reside in the country, not taking out insurance can result in sanctions as well. As soon as a contract is agreed, a previously uninsured person can be obliged to pay a supplementary penalty fee if they delayed taking out insurance longer than three months after their arrival in the country. In consequence of it being both a duty and right to take out insurance, Rüefli & Hügli propose the following goal:

> all undocumented migrants who are legally obliged to have health insurance [...] have taken out insurance and have the same access to care providers and medical services, within the scope of basic health provision, as insured people with legal residence. (2011:19)[1]

Still, this goal is not shared by all political players in the country. In 2016, Ulrich Giezendanner, a member of the right wing Schweizerische Volkspartei (SVP), began a parliamentary initiative asking that undocumented migrants be denied the right to obtain health insurance. The initiative was taken up by the National Council's Commission for Social Security and Health, and will now be discussed in the National Council on the basis of a vague idea according to which healthcare for undocumented migrants would be provided by a state-financed organization. The Federal Council, on the other hand, recommends the Council reject the motion (SGK 2018).

Policies also vary from canton to canton. Thus, until 2012, it was not clear whether failed asylum seekers had to be granted insurance by the cantons, who are also in charge of the implementation of the laws governing asylum. In addition, a few atypical cantons, like Vaud and Geneva, have adopted policies that allow for the provision of special services to vulnerable populations, which include undocumented migrants. Financing is granted via cantons and municipalities, and the functioning of the services is sustained by tight links between administrations, NGOs and service providers (see Marks-Sultan et al. 2016; Piccoli 2016:17). In the majority of other cantons, including the region on which this study focusses, there are no special arrangements and the national policy is the only one on which service providers and patients can rely.

---

1   Any quotes from literature not originally in English have been translated by the author and will be given in the original language in the footnotes. Here: 'Alle versicherungspflichtigen Sans Papiers [...] sind krankenversichert und haben denselben Zugang zu denselben Leistungserbringern und Leistungen des medizinischen Grundleistungskatalogs wie versicherte Personen mit legalem Aufenthalt'.

Detailing the variations between the different policies that regulate healthcare for undocumented migrants demonstrates their differences in content, time and space. Thus, policies shape very specific contexts of care for undocumented migrants in a certain time and place. Local studies, as proposed by this report, can shed light on these contexts.

... and practices

This section will look at how specific healthcare policies shape healthcare practices — meaning the concrete situations of accessing, giving and receiving healthcare — in the case of undocumented migrants. As we will see, restrictive, ambiguous and quickly changing policies cause difficulties in relation to the practical delivery of healthcare, while even in inclusive environments, significant barriers remain. Again, we will turn first to the situation in Europe, and then focus on the Swiss context.

As a result of ambiguous and varying healthcare policies, it can be difficult for undocumented migrants to know what kind of healthcare they are entitled to. For instance, Poduval et al. (2015) analysed patients' and professionals' experiences, collected in interviews conducted at a Doctors of the World surgery in London. They report that undocumented migrants are insufficiently aware of their rights. For example, they do not know they are entitled to register with a general practitioner. As a result, undocumented migrants tend to prefer emergency departments. Similarly, Sigona & Hughes (2012:35) state that while most of the undocumented children they studied had a general practitioner, many of the parents did not clearly understand whether or not adults were entitled to the same access.

Lack of knowledge can also be a difficulty for healthcare professionals. In Spain, migrants had difficulties in accessing and obtaining healthcare that were partially due to confusion about regional implementation after the change in the law in 2012, which left healthcare professionals with unclear information about what level of healthcare they were still allowed to deliver to undocumented migrants (Roura et al. 2015). Falla et al. (2016) use the example of treatment for hepatitis B and C to demonstrate the diversity of beliefs among professionals about undocumented migrants' entitlement to care.

As a result of restrictive policies, healthcare services are underused. Referring patients to hospital is difficult if secondary care is not accessible, especially if it is not easy to decide whether an operation is urgent or not (Sigona & Hughes 2012:39). There is room for alternative strategies, such as 'borrowing medical cards and resorting to emergency care for non-urgent conditions' (Roura et al. 2015) but also 'self-medication and contacting doctors in home countries' (Biswas et al. 2011).

Undocumented migrants need special knowledge to access some types of healthcare, which is provided by informal networks often organized by NGOs in parallel systems (Huschke 2014). Drawing on the work of Pierre Bourdieu, Huschke shows how social capital is a critical, fragile and transformative factor in this endeavour. Biswas et al. (2011), through interviews with undocumented migrants and emergency room nurses, show that receiving help from Danish citizens proves to be a central strategy when it comes to accessing healthcare. Similarly in Milan, a city in the Lombardy region of Italy where policies are rather restrictive, the time between entering the country and first being seen by a healthcare professional can be reduced by 30% if a person can rely on strong social ties, as a network analysis by Devillanova (2008) shows.

Difficulties in achieving access are also reported in countries where more inclusive policies are in place. Before the national policy changed in Spain in 2012, the migrant population was granted wide-reaching access to healthcare for about three decades. But Vasquez et al. still see 'inequalities in health among this population which signal social inequalities in access to care' (2013:237).

Similar problems can be seen in France, despite Laranché's belief that 'it could be said to hold one of the most liberal and progressive healthcare systems in the world' (2012:858). Laranché demonstrates through participant observation that social stigmatization, precarious living conditions and suspicion towards immigrants prevent undocumented migrants from accessing healthcare in France. By drawing on theories influenced by Michel Foucault and Judith Butler, Laranché argues that 'intangible factors' affect both undocumented migrants and healthcare providers. Stigmatizing discourse and prejudice shape the views of both sides about what kind of care undocumented migrants deserve.

As a consequence, problems can arise in areas where access is not in question. In the UK for example, even though access is granted for primary care,

> in the majority of cases individuals registered very soon after their arrival in the UK and while having some form of residence status. (Sigona & Hughes 2012:35)

Later, patients often travel long distances to visit their general practitioners. Drawing on Laranché, such a situation could be seen as partially the result of discourse and practice, leaving undocumented migrants without the courage to visit a more conveniently located healthcare provider once they have lost their legal status.

In Switzerland, there are about fourteen service providers delivering care to undocumented migrants in the country (Altenburg 2012). Most of the providers are NGOs and charitable institutions (see also Bilger et al. 2011; Weiss 2015). Thus, in a manner similar to other countries, it seems likely that there is a discrepancy between the legal entitlement to insurance with associated care, and the actual delivery of healthcare to undocumented migrants through NGOs and charities. For example, turning their attention to one specific aspect of medical provision, namely pregnancy care and prevention, Wolff & Epiney (2008) show that in Geneva undocumented migrants use such services less than legal residents. For instance, undocumented migrants consulted for an initial pregnancy visit four weeks later than legal residents, and while among the latter only 2% had never had a cervical smear test, this was the case for 18% of the undocumented women.

Reasons for this discrepancy can be found in Bilger et al. (2011) who report healthcare professionals asserting that undocumented migrants lack trust in health service organizations and experience difficulties paying for healthcare and/or insurance. Weidtmann (2015) concentrates on the barriers that hinder people from taking out insurance and interviews two undocumented migrants alongside employees of NGOs and social services. She identifies financial and administrative challenges as the main obstacles. These difficulties are further exacerbated by problems with language, a lack of knowledge about the system, and fear.

In the light of these studies it is not surprising that reviews (Woodward et al. 2013; De Vito et al. 2016) and studies investigating the practices of several European countries (Dauvin 2012) report that even though in many cases legal *entitlement* may be in place, this does 'not correspond with *access* to care' (Woodward et al. 2013:826). Barriers for undocumented migrants within the healthcare system can be attributed to external resource constraints–such as lack of transportation or limited healthcare capacity–or to discrimination and excessive bureaucratic requirements. On the patients' side, undocumented migrants avoid seeking care because of communication problems, financial restrictions, or out of fear of deportation (Hacker et al. 2015). Access to mental health resources is a particularly critical issue (Strassmayr et al. 2012).

Furthermore, qualitative studies, like those by Poduval et al. (2015), Biswas et al. (2011), Laranché (2012) or Huschke (2014), take into account the views of professionals and patients, and highlight promising ways to further examine healthcare practices in relation to concepts including politics, power, communication and social institutions.

In my third chapter, I shall demonstrate how a local study such as mine can address the need for 'research which focuses on the treatment of migrants with particular emphasis on the interplay between the various providers of care' (Achermann 2006:202)[2] within Switzerland, whilst simultaneously drawing on the research approach of the above-mentioned qualitative studies, linking healthcare practice to concepts stemming from ethnography and sociology.

Undocumented migrants' health

Having discussed the ways in which we can understand the policies and practices that shape healthcare for undocumented migrants, the question remains: what kind of health challenges do they face? Recent attempts to shed light on these challenges call into question established ways of thinking about migrants as a homogeneous group of healthy or ill bodies with well-defined characteristics.

One area of migrant healthcare that has traditionally received a great deal of attention concerns communicable diseases and reproductive health. In a colonial and postcolonial context, this research and policy

---

2   'Forschung im Bereich Migration, Prekarität und Gesundheit zum Umgang mit betroffenen MigrantInnen, wobei das Zusammenspiel von verschiedenen leistungserbringenden Akteuren besonders beachtet werden sollte'.

focus often aligns with the idea of migrants as diseased bodies that might bring danger to a 'native' population. At the same time, this research tradition shows how Public Health, a discipline that as a whole strongly focuses on communicable diseases, turns its attention also to migrants' health, and thus to a population that is often overlooked (Bivins 2015). This research emphasis holds true for undocumented migrants in Switzerland: Bodenmann et al. (2009) show that out of 125 screened undocumented migrants, 19.2% had a latent tuberculosis infection. Sebo et al. (2011) and Casillas et al. (2015) examine the sexual and reproductive health behaviour of undocumented women and discover low levels of contraceptive use and correspondingly high rates of unplanned pregnancies.

A second important research focus when it comes to migrants' health is expressed by the concept of the so-called 'healthy migrant paradox' (Domnich 2012). Using this idea, researchers attempt to explain the lower mortality rates among immigrants compared to local populations by asserting that, typically, migration is 'working migration' and so only people of generally good health choose to, are chosen to or are able to migrate.

However, there is more to the picture. For instance, a growing body of studies shows that migrants' health generally deteriorates quickly after their arrival (Gushulak 2007; Woodward et al. 2013), calling into question both the concept of 'the migrant as a travelling disease' and the healthy migrant paradox.

Further, an exclusive focus on communicable diseases might overlook other important health issues. For example, an analysis of drug prescription to undocumented migrants by a Milanese NGO shows that non-communicable chronic diseases appear to be prevalent among undocumented migrants (Fiorini et al. 2016). Mental health seems to be particularly affected: subjective perception of health in undocumented migrants is significantly worse than amongst a comparative sample of legal residents (Kuehne et al. 2015). From a medical point of view, another study found that 47.6% of the twenty-one undocumented migrants who were interviewed presented symptoms of anxiety and/or depression (Heeren et al. 2014).

Interestingly, residential status appears to have a causal impact on mental health (Martinez et al. 2015; Heeren et al. 2014; Sigona & Hughes 2012). Furthermore, and perhaps unsurprisingly, there is also a link between barriers to healthcare, constructed through restrictive healthcare policies or practices, and an increased risk to the health of undocumented migrants. A systematic review identified thirty quantitative and qualitative studies and policy analyses drawing links between anti-immigration policies, barriers to healthcare access, and health status (Martinez et al. 2015). For example, a study conducted at a Berlin clinic for undocumented migrants showed that for all of the most common problems — chiefly pregnancy, chronic illness and mental health conditions — patients presented late and with significant complications due to barriers to accessing healthcare (Castaneda 2009).

Sigona & Hughes in turn inform us that *The Confidential Enquiry into Maternal and Child Health* in 2007 found that about 20% of deaths directly or indirectly related to pregnancy occurred in women with poor or no antenatal care. The authors propose that

> one of the main deterrents to accessing maternity care may be the policy of charging 'non ordinarily resident' patients introduced in 2004. (Signoa & Hughes 2012:34)

It is thus not very surprising that Cerri et al. (2017), analysing the prescription of psychiatric medications, found that prescription rates were higher for Italian natives than for undocumented migrants, despite the well-documented phenomenon of mental health issues being more prevalent amongst the latter. Exacerbation of certain health-related problems and underuse of health services go hand in hand.

Thus, the research focus has now shifted from the focus on transmittable diseases and the healthy migrant paradox to the idea that a person's legal status and the conditions in their country of arrival are a social determinant of their health, a social factor that causally influences health outcomes (Rechel et al. 2013; Castaneda et al. 2015).

The retelling of the undocumented migrants' stories will draw on these insights by situating them within an analytical framework that allows the careful exploration and retracing of causal links between social institutions, legal arrangements and undocumented migrants' health.

3. Telling stories about healthcare for undocumented migrants

This chapter discusses the context in which the material for this report was collected and will therefore give the reader a first look at the NGO. Next, the theoretical perspective taken to analyse these materials will be outlined, before bringing both strands together to introduce the reader to the undocumented migrants' stories, as told in Chapters Four to Six.

Collecting materials at and around the NGO

All patients interviewed were accessed via the same NGO, already mentioned in the introduction. Of course, this excludes undocumented migrants who might not need or know about the NGO (Fleischmann et al. 2015; Fiorini et al. 2016 discuss similar limitations). Finally, patients who might have had negative experiences with the NGO, and therefore no longer attend, could not be interviewed.

Eight patients were interviewed. Their ages ranged between early twenties and late forties, an age span common among those accessing Swiss NGOs in general (Bilger et al. 2011:43). Interviews were conducted in German, French, and English, lasting from twenty to ninety minutes.

Professionals were approached directly, via the NGO or by 'snowballing', or word of mouth. Ten professionals were interviewed, with discussions lasting between thirty and ninety minutes. Two interviewees were employed by the NGO, four were volunteers related to the NGO, two worked at a public hospital, one was an insurance

 https://doi.org/10.11647/OBP.0139.03

company employee and one worked for an NGO caring for HIV-positive undocumented migrants.

The protection of interviewees is an important issue, especially when they are undocumented migrants. In order to ensure anonymity, all interviewees are given pseudonyms here and all statements translated into English. Furthermore, as Switzerland is a small country with even smaller regional structures, the exact location of the NGO is kept confidential. It is only relevant to know that this NGO is located in one of the regions where there is no specific regional policy concerning healthcare for undocumented migrants.

The NGO takes care of about 130 patients per year. Using the estimated number of undocumented migrants in the catchment area, it can be extrapolated that the NGO sees approximately 2%-4% of the population of undocumented migrants yearly. About one third of the patients only go to the NGO once. Another third attend episodically, and the remaining third visit regularly. The head of this NGO is Julia, the nurse we encountered in the introduction, and she carries out operational work together with a second nurse, Melanie. All other professionals at the facility are volunteers and we will encounter them as we hear the undocumented migrants' stories.

The NGO offers drop-in consultation hours, as well as consultations by appointment. Still, it should not be thought of as a doctor's office, as David, a volunteering general practitioner, says:

> Well, you see, there are many things we can't offer. I mean, we now have an ECG [electrocardiogram]. But we have no spirometer, we can't fully examine people's hearing and so on. We don't have our own lab. We're only open three half days a week. I don't really give injections; we don't really have the equipment.

In part, the limited staffing and scant equipment in the NGO are due to financial restrictions. On the other hand, this sparseness is also intentional, as the aim of the NGO is to serve as a point of 'triage into regular care' as Julia says. Echoing the goal stated by Hügli & Rüefli (2011) to provide all undocumented migrants with healthcare via insurance, Julia's statement refers to the idea of 'integrational inclusion' (Stichweh 2007:8), in other words, of bringing all patients together into the same system, rather than separating the healthcare of legal residents and undocumented migrants.

Healthcare for undocumented migrants as a process

The following section will introduce the reader to the way in which this study retells and makes sense of its material, gathered at and around the NGO. In order to gain meaningful insights from the interviews, a processual understanding of 'undocumentedness' and healthcare is needed. This idea stems as much from the literature discussed above as from the material gathered for this work, which reveals individual experiences that are in constant flux, in relation both to the person's changing legal status and to the healthcare they receive. It is important for the analytical approach to be tailored to the nature of the material; otherwise the most interesting aspects might be lost (Glaser & Strauss 2006 [1967]; Corbin & Strauss 1990).

The concept of 'access', although widely used in medical literature, is not very suitable for a processual approach. In the above-mentioned studies, 'access' is used in a rather broad and unspecific way, sometimes focusing on rights and systemic arrangements for access (PICUM 2007; Biffl et al. 2012; Björngren-Cuadra 2012; Biswas et al. 2012), at other times concentrating on concrete administrative aspects (Poduval 2012), or on the actual use of healthcare services, while at other times addressing and linking several of these at once (Laranché 2012).

Levesque et al. (2013) expand the concept of access to its extreme, encompassing the entire process from the moment the need for healthcare is identified, to what happens in the course of finding a healthcare provider, and even including the outcomes of healthcare interventions. Although this brings them close to a processual approach, the authors overstretch the definition of access, describing it as:

> a way of approaching, reaching or entering a place, as the right or opportunity to reach, use or visit. (Levesque et al. 2013 citing the Canadian Oxford Dictionary)

'Access' is thus a term that might not fully express the complexity of obtaining healthcare without reaching the limits of its plausible definition.

Furthermore, the concept of access lacks a suitable counterpart to express the idea that once access is achieved, it can also be lost again.

Talking about barriers also gives the impression that once they are overcome, one has achieved access to healthcare for good. Recent critics of the concept have argued that it would make more sense to talk about 'healthcare pathways' rather than 'access as a one-off event' (Hanenssgen & Proochista 2017). Another suggested approach is to frame access as a process of 'candidacy', characterized by negotiations between individuals and health services, where these negotiations define 'peoples' eligibility for medical attention and intervention' (Dixon-Woods et al. 2006).

One framework that incorporates the need for a processual and interaction-oriented approach, one fitted to an analysis of the complex and dynamic processes that affect healthcare for undocumented migrants, is the sociological dyad of inclusion and exclusion. There are three different research traditions in sociology relating to this dyad (Stichweh 2007). In France, the discussion started with Émile Durkheim and addresses questions of social cohesion. This way of thinking has entered the public debate, engaging authors such as Michel Foucault and Pierre Bourdieu. The British theory of the welfare state has been dealing with this concept since about 1960, when Thomas Humphrey Marshall first introduced it. In a German context, it is related to Niklas Luhmann's system theory (Luhmann 1991), which, in turn, engages critically with Talcott Parsons's sociological work. Rudolph Stichweh continues this tradition and asserts that

> the two terms, inclusion and exclusion, designate the way in which social systems relate to persons in their environment. (2007:2)[1]

In this framework, social systems are conceptualised as not only consisting of communication but also as being created, stabilized and changed by communication, and in this sense the approach is constructivist.

A person's inclusion in the social system is dependent on the extent to which he or she is addressed by the communication that constitutes that system (Luhmann 1997:620). Inclusion should thus be differentiated from concepts such as integration. Inclusion is about a 'connection to

---

1   'Mit den beiden Begriffen Inklusion und Exklusion [wird] die Art und Weise bezeichnet, in der Sozialsysteme sich auf ihre personale Umwelt beziehen'.

contexts of communication' and not about the 'integration of people through shared norms and values' (Nassehi & Nollmann 1997:394).[2]

According to this theoretical approach, interactions (e.g. oral communication) as well as organizations and functional social realms form social systems. Interactions can happen within the frame of organizations and/or functional systems. The migrants' stories describe their inclusion within organizations such as the NGO, an insurance company, a hospital, or similar. In order to be included in these organizations, specific types of communication are necessary. A hospital might, for example, set up communications between an administrative employee and a potential patient. Furthermore, within organizations, instances of communication might relate to various functional systems. For example, the payment of insurance is an instance of communication belonging to the economic system, while a patient's interaction with a nurse is an act of communication situated within the healthcare system (Luhmann 1991; 1997). The present study thus examines inclusion in and exclusion from communication in the healthcare system itself, for example in the interaction between healthcare professionals and patients. However this book also investigates systems and organizations that are not part of the healthcare system but are linked to it, such as communication taking place in an insurance hub or in the adminstrative department of a hospital. When I discuss inclusion in or exclusion from healthcare, I am also referring to these organizations and systems.

This approach also allows a closer look at the 'links between different forms of inclusion' (Bommes & Tacke 2001:63).[3] One might, for example, ask how inclusion in a system of insurance is connected to inclusion in, or exclusion from, a hospital. This in turn enables a re-examination of the idea that a person's legal status influences both their healthcare and their health. Finally, one can gain insight into the benefits and drawbacks that patients and professionals ascribe to inclusion and exclusion, and therefore build up detailed characterizations of the inclusion or exclusion of undocumented migrants in or from communication related to healthcare.

---

2   'Anbindung [...] an Kommunikationszusammenhänge' und nicht etwa um eine 'Integration von Menschen durch geteilte Normen und Werte'.
3   'Zusammenhänge zwischen verschiedenen Inklusionsformen zu stellen'.

In addition, inclusion and exclusion are not fixed states, but are created or undone during every moment of communication in which a specific person is either addressed, or not. As Stichweh notes:

> First and foremost, we must emphasize that inclusion and exclusion are characterized as events. They are executed as operations. (2007:3)[4]

The dyad of inclusion and exclusion thus allows insight into the undocumented migrants' stories, causing us to ask at each stage whether the communication taking place includes or excludes undocumented migrants from healthcare.

At this point, some remarks on the concept of health might be appropriate. A universal definition is far out of reach (see Lewis 2001 for an overview). Existing formulations range from the description of health simply as an absence of illness to much broader ideas, such as that of the World Health Organization (WHO), which defines health as 'a state of complete physical, mental and social well-being' (WHO 1992). Furthermore, as medical anthropology shows, ideas about health and well-being need to be understood within their social contexts (Pool & Geissler 2005), calling into question the possibility of a uniform definition. For the purposes of this study, the definition of what health means and how encompassing the concept might be was left to interviewees. The aim in so doing was to trace common patterns in undocumented migrants' conceptions of health and wellbeing.

With its turn to inclusion and exclusion as a conceptual framework, this section has given us a suitable approach for analysing stories about healthcare for undocumented migrants. The concept of communication, which structures various social systems and enables the inclusion or exclusion of undocumented migrants from those systems, gives the analysis a clear focus. What exactly inclusion and exclusion means for undocumented migrants, and how their dynamics affect migrants' health, will be discussed in the collected stories. Indeed, the main analytical focus of this study is the investigation of the dynamics of inclusion and exclusion from communication in the healthcare system and related to the healthcare system.

---

4   'Es ist zunächst der Ereignischarakter von Inklusion und Exklusion und damit zugleich der operative Vollzug von Inklusionen und Exklusionen zu betonen'.

Core moments of inclusion

Before turning to the undocumented migrants' stories, let us look at how they are linked to the conceptual framework of inclusion and exclusion.

The interviews with patients form the focal point of the study, and each of them is examined to discern the event that the interviewees describe as the core moment of their inclusion in healthcare. These moments are recounted by the patients in a spontaneous, detailed and animated manner, as they recall the incidents that helped them to address their health issues in a way that they define as good, or at least satisfactory. These specific moments are therefore at the very heart of this study. The following pages contain groups of interviews that describe similar core moments of inclusion.

Some of the undocumented migrants experienced periods of complete exclusion from healthcare or went without treatment for specific conditions before reaching their core moment of inclusion. These moments therefore mark turning points after periods of struggle–some lasting months, others years–as they coped with health issues more or less on their own. On the other hand, some of the patients identified persistent difficulties even after this core moment had been reached. These stories were more complex and involved, depending on how lengthy and challenging the period before the core moment had been and the size of the difficulties that remained. The order of the stories within the chapters has been chosen by taking this growing complexity into account, so every story will reveal further moments of exclusion, but also further strategies for inclusion.

The tables below provide an overview of the following three chapters, introducing the individual patients and the main healthcare issues they report, both before and after their core moment of inclusion.

One such moment related by Suzanne (Figure 6) concerns her progress with settling in. This core moment of inclusion stands at the centre of Chapter Four, and it is introduced with some notes about undocumented migrants' living conditions.

A second core moment of inclusion, described by four of the interviewees (Figure 7), is their experience of obtaining healthcare at the NGO and its network. Their stories are related in Chapter Five, starting with some general information about the NGO.

Patient	Major issues before core moment of inclusion	Core moment of inclusion	Remaining major issues after core moment of inclusion
Suzanne	Lacking direction, Suzanne misses her family and has few working opportunities.	Suzanne finds a job, housing and friends, she can support her family back home.	No major issues.

Fig. 6 Settling in as core moment of inclusion.

Patient	Major issues before core moment of inclusion	Core moment of inclusion	Remaining major issues after core moment of inclusion
Béatrice	No major issues.	Béatrice gets treatment for her dental problems through the NGO's network.	No major issues.
Peter	Peter does not obtain care for his mental health issues for about one and a half years. Healthcare is lacking continuity.	He gets help at the NGO and therapy for his mental health problems through the NGO's network.	Continuity of care is still not fully ensured while Peter remains under the constant threat of being deported.
Maria	Maria has had no access to any care for about seven years; a broad spectrum of symptoms have emerged during this time.	She is treated for depression, anaemia, low iron levels and high blood pressure by the NGO and its network.	Lacking an income and thus an insurance policy, Maria cannot get surgery to treat her fibroid. She fears a negative outcome of the procedures concerning her legal status.
Jonathan	With untreated diabetes and without opportunities for employment, Jonathan remains completely excluded from healthcare for about a year. This period is interrupted once by an asylum process.	Being treated for diabetes by the NGO's network, Jonathan also gets some help in terms of housing and food.	Due to Jonathan's very precarious living conditions, all attempts at inclusion remain partial and precarious.

Fig. 7 Getting in touch with the NGO and its network as a core moment of inclusion.

For the three remaining patients interviewed, Anna, Fanny and Nicolas (Figure 8), taking out insurance was their core moment of inclusion. Their stories are told in Chapter Six, introduced by some additional notes concerning insurance for undocumented migrants.

When looking at this overview of the patients' perspectives, it should not be forgotten that inclusion and exclusion are social relations. The undocumented migrants are not the only actors to consider; there are also the healthcare professionals, embedded in their roles, organizations and rules. Their point of view is important to help us understand and contextualise the struggles and successes of undocumented migrants in tending to their health and healthcare needs.

Patient	Major issues before core moment of inclusion	Core moment of inclusion	Remaining major issues after core moment of inclusion
Anna	No major issues.	The acquisition of insurance allows Anna's breast cancer to be treated.	Due to very precarious working conditions, Anna has great difficulties paying for the insurance.
Fanny	With only one remaining kidney, Fanny is completely excluded from healthcare for about eight years. This period is interrupted once by an asylum process, during which she can give birth while being in touch with healthcare professionals.	Taking out insurance leads to continuous care during Fanny's second pregnancy.	Paying for the insurance remains an issue. Fanny's children are still uninsured.
Nicolas	Without insurance or contact with the NGO for about seven years, Nicolas has to deal with an accident at work and eye problems.	After taking out insurance Nicolas can get eye surgery and is protected in case of future accidents at work.	Paying for the insurance is an ongoing issue for Nicolas. His biggest problem is his residential status.

Fig. 8 Reaching out for insurance as a core moment of inclusion.

While I focus on the stories of patients, there are other actors or organisations which reoccur throughout the various narratives and chapters. In Suzanne's story about settling in, for example, we find the first reference to the NGO. Jonathan's story, in which the NGO plays the most important role, also brings issues about insurance into the picture. And the NGO remains an important place for undocumented migrants who have obtained insurance, as we will see in Chapter Six.

4. Settling in

.

This chapter describes the case of Suzanne, a young and healthy undocumented migrant whose core moment of inclusion was brought about by finding a job, a social circle and a place to live — in other words, by settling in. This case also tells us many things about the preconditions of inclusion in healthcare.

In any given year, about 2%-4% of the total population of the area under scrutiny attend the NGO. There are certainly undocumented migrants in the area who are in good health and never attend the NGO, perhaps not even knowing of its existence. Thus, the story in this chapter is probably common to other young and healthy undocumented migrants, who, as the head of the NGO confirms, make up a significant portion of the population. Over time though, a greater percentage of undocumented migrants might attend an NGO. Indeed, Achermann et al. (2006:147) state in their study that out of eighteen undocumented migrants, only six had never seen a doctor, those mostly being people who had only been undocumented for a short time.

As in the case of Suzanne, it is estimated that most (Bilger et al. 2011:51), meaning around 80%-90% of undocumented migrants, are uninsured (Rüefli & Hügli 2011:24). The explanation for this allows us to take a closer look at undocumented migrants' economic and legal situations (see also Achermann et al. 2006).

In reference to their economic situation, the head of the NGO estimates that an undocumented migrant in the region might be able to earn around CHF 800 to 1500 a month, while some might have no income whatsoever. She therefore broadly confirms the estimates of those authors who suggest that undocumented migrants in various

 https://doi.org/10.11647/OBP.0139.04

Swiss regions earn between CHF 600 and 2000 a month (Chiementi et al. 2003:38; Valli 2003:34; Anlaufstelle für Sans-Papiers 2004:11; Achermann et al. 2006:113).

In order to contextualise the affordability of health insurance on such an income, we can use the example of a hypothetical person living in Zurich. If we go to www.comparis.ch, a website that offers comparisons between insurance policies, and look for basic insurance with accident cover for a twenty-seven year old, we find that the cheapest plan and the lowest annual excess of CHF 300 will result in a premium of CHF 395 per month (as of 16 March 2017). This constitutes roughly 26% to 49% of an undocumented migrant's monthly income. Furthermore, if care is needed, 10% of the cost, up to a limit of CHF 700 (the so-called 'deductible') has to be paid out of pocket.

Those living in reduced economic circumstances might have access to premium subsidies in Switzerland. For a moment, leave aside the question of whether and how such subsidies are obtainable for undocumented migrants (see Rüefli & Hügli 2011:30ff). As of 2017 a twenty-seven year old person in Zürich can claim a maximum subsidy of CHF 1,644 per annum (Sozialversicherungsanstalt des Kantons Zürich 2017). This would mean a monthly premium of CHF 258, which would still constitute 17% to 32% of the monthly income of an undocumented migrant in the area under discussion.

By comparison, Swiss citizens without children and a low to moderate monthly gross income of CHF 2,500 to 5,000 (a Swiss citizen in 2015 had a median monthly gross income of CHF 6,500) spend 8% to 11% of this on health insurance (Lampart et al. 2016). The goal set by the revision of the insurance law in 2012 was to freeze the proportion at 8% (Lampart et al. 2015). Of course, these limits apply to people who are otherwise included in basic legal and social security schemes, with employment contracts that factor in provision for sick pay or notice periods, unemployment insurance, maternity insurance and the like.

To choose an annual excess of CHF 2,500, which would result in a lower premium, is too great a risk for an undocumented migrant. A patient would have to put aside CHF 2,500 on top of CHF 700 deductible, which represents at least two and at worst four months' salary. In case of non-payment, the patient risks being exposed as undocumented, a problem that also arises in the UK with the Memorandum of Understanding on

Data-Sharing Inquiry that allows data sharing between the NHS and the Home Office (UK Parliament 2018).

Fear of deportation often prevents undocumented migrants from taking out insurance in the first place. Any contact whatsoever with an organization that might be related to the state is avoided. Consequently, it is highly improbable that undocumented migrants would give their address to an insurance company — but if a person does not hold a current Swiss health insurance policy, they must provide proof of residence when applying, which is usually handed out by the municipality. An undocumented migrant lacks this proof. As stated by Patricia, the insurance employee whom I interviewed:

> *A normal administrator just looks at the dossier, is it complete [...] and is there a confirmation of registration from the municipality. If not, he checks with the municipality.*

This cross-checking with the municipality actually violates data protection rules (KVG 84ff; see also Hüegli & Rüfli 2011:32). In most cases, if clients simply forget to enclose the confirmation, or postpone its submission, this violation has no negative consequences. In the case of undocumented migrants however it can lead to deportation. In addition, a bank account is needed in order to organize financial transactions related to the insurance policy. But to open a bank account, one needs proof of residency in Switzerland.

Given all these issues, insurance is not a reliable vehicle for inclusion and it is at this juncture in Suzanne's case, as with many undocumented migrants, that the NGO enters the picture. We are about to be introduced to Julia, the head of the NGO whom I mentioned earlier, as well as a general physician called David, a gynaecologist named Patrick, and another general physician with a specialization in ultrasound who volunteers at the NGO.

Suzanne: 'Now, it's just fine'

The interview with Suzanne takes place as she attends the NGO on a drop-in morning. Suzanne is in her twenties and has been living as an undocumented migrant in Switzerland for about four years now. Generally, Suzanne seems to feel that she is in good health. During the interview, she mentions several times that she does not consider herself able to contribute much to my project: on the one hand, her linguistic skills in our common language are slightly limited, on the other, Suzanne repeatedly states that at the moment, she's very well. However, it is precisely because of this latter circumstance that Suzanne can give valuable insights regarding the question of what health means to an undocumented migrant and how undocumented migrants try to care for their health, despite limited resources.

Asked about her story, she says of her first two years in Switzerland:

> *For me it was rather terrible and I missed my family a lot, and my daughter, and I cried a lot, almost every day.*

The difficulty of leaving one's family behind will also appear in other patients' stories. Here, at the very beginning of Suzanne's narrative, we encounter the idea that there might be specific conditions in the life of undocumented migrants that could bring out particular health issues, such as the risk of mental illness brought about or exacerbated by isolation. Julia says that many of the health problems suffered by undocumented migrants are related to poor living and housing conditions, risky jobs, fear of being caught, missing their family and dependency on the goodwill of others for most common necessities.

But Julia immediately contrasts these difficulties with the cleverness, good language skills and independence of some undocumented migrants and refers to them as 'survival artists'. Similarly, David, the general practitioner volunteering at the NGO attests to their 'virtuosity' in handling daily life. In a similar vein, Suzanne states, just after talking about how she had cried almost every day: 'And yes, now it's just fine'.

With these statements, we can see that it is important for both caregivers and the patients themselves to see that their status as undocumented migrants does not mean they are simply victims, at the mercy of circumstance, but they are also as active agents, able to control their own lives. We will see on several occasions that it is important for undocumented migrants to have agency, and to achieve inclusion in healthcare themselves, rather than having to refer to and depend on others.

But then, how did things become 'fine' for Suzanne after two years of struggle? How did she overcome the pain of leaving her family and especially her daughter behind? She says:

> *And then I got to know other women here and, yes, these women helped me so much. With work and so on.* [Interviewer: Other women from your home country?] *Yes, yes. I know two or three women. But now they have become good friends of mine* [laughs]. *And these women also work here. And I also work a bit more as a cleaner and sometimes I mind children.*

We can see here that getting in touch with the local diaspora and finding work are decisive in helping Suzanne to live a 'fine' life. Indeed, Suzanne came to Switzerland with another woman from her country. This connection, together with her relationships with other compatriots in the area, gave her opportunities to find work. In addition, Suzanne learned one of the Swiss national languages.

As a result of her employment, Suzanne is able to support her daughter back home. This also helps her to address the pressures that accompany her status as an undocumented migrant. Inclusion in healthcare often affects more people than just the individual concerned. For Suzanne, for instance, her inclusion also helps her to care for her relatives who stayed at home. As we will see, the ability to support those 'back home' is also important for other undocumented migrants.

Finally, the NGO provides Suzanne with a place that 'I can come to when I have something' and thus helps her to create the conditions for healthy living, most importantly stability. One of her friends told her about it and at first she did not attend, as she did not see any need. Then, her friend told her it would be good to have a gynaecological check-up so she dropped in for the first time, her friend translating. The day of the interview is her third visit. She is here because of a cough and also for her ear, in which she has been experiencing hearing loss for several years and which is now aching and oozes liquid. She will be sent to the NGO's network for her ear to be examined, and we will hear more about this network later on. For her, inclusion in healthcare is the knowledge that should she have some more serious issues, she has a place to go to.

The gynaecologist volunteering at the Access Point, Patrick, offers the professional's point of view concerning routine gynaecological check-ups. He states:

> Here I don't notice much about their background, except that there's sometimes a language problem. Other than that, it's like it was when I was working as a gynaecologist in [a Swiss hospital].

Both he and the ultrasound expert state that, among the patients they have seen so far, they would not have been able to tell an undocumented migrant from a citizen.

Knowing that the NGO exists and (more importantly) finding a few friends and some work all allowed Suzanne to secure and maintain good health.

It is important to her that she can help her daughter and thus address her loneliness and sadness, problems that arise from her undocumented status. Her inclusion in healthcare also enables her to care for those left behind. Health, and inclusion in healthcare, are thus embedded into, and dependent on, social relations.

Suzanne has made a life for herself. She has found a secure base and thus she can be an active agent in relation to her own health. This autonomy contributes to her wellbeing. According to the professionals whose experiences are related in this chapter, the inclusion of undocumented migrants in healthcare can be quite unproblematic and does not necessarily require specific skills.

5. The NGO and its network

In this chapter, we will encounter patients who, unlike Suzanne, have experienced more serious health issues and for whom the NGO and its network have proved to be important for their inclusion in healthcare as well as for maintaining their general health.

About a third of the patients attend the NGO regularly and another third use the service sporadically. While Béatrice, whom we will encounter first, probably belongs to the latter category, Peter, Maria and Jonathan are long-term regular patients. During their stay in Switzerland, they have also experienced periods of partial or total exclusion from healthcare. Their experiences during these times may well reflect those of patients who have some health issues, but do not know about the NGO.

As in the previous chapter, a very important factor that enables inclusion in healthcare–insurance–is not an active part of these stories. In the case of Béatrice, the dental care she needs is not covered by insurance. Furthermore, her story is the first to reveal that the emergency services are another potential point of inclusion that is often bypassed. Béatrice's statements will be complemented by the perspectives of Andrew, an administrative employee, and a doctor, Carl, who work in the emergency service of a public hospital. Béatrice's story offers more information about the interactions of both the individual patient and the NGO with professionals in the NGO's network.

For Peter and Jonathan, insurance is a background issue. They have insurance, but only because others have taken on the entire administrative and financial burden of obtaining it for them. Again, the NGO and its network are their most important points of reference.

 https://doi.org/10.11647/OBP.0139.05

Jonathan's story highlights, for the first time, the role the NGO plays in taking out insurance for a patient. We will also see what this process involves from the perspective of an insurance employee, Patricia. Furthermore, through an interview with Caroline, a diabetes counsellor within the NGO's network, we will examine in more detail how the professionals in this network contribute to Jonathan's inclusion in healthcare. Finally, for Maria it is the care at the NGO and within its network that proved to be her most important moment of inclusion, because for her, insurance is financially out of reach.

Concerning uninsured patients, it is important to note that, as Julia puts it, the NGO has a 'relationship of dependency'with the professionals in its network. Indeed, they often work extra hours of their own accord and for reduced pay. It is not easy to build up such a network and all the volunteers have particular motivations for their work. For example, David, the general practitioner volunteering at the NGO, states that he has often worked with socially vulnerable patients in the past. The gynaecologist and the ultrasound expert whom we met during Suzanne's story have both worked in hospitals in so-called developing countries. The head of the NGO describes her work with the network as time-consuming. She always needs to arrange

> *very binding deals, but with individuals, because we don't really have any* [formal] *agreements.*

This is echoed by Melanie, the other nurse working at the NGO:

> *We're always dependent on there being people with a good heart, or someone who feels, yes, we really must help these people.*

Béatrice: 'They always find a solution'

Béatrice is a woman in her thirties, who has been living in Switzerland for about four years. She initially portrays her life as an 'adventure', but a few moments later, she starts to muse that God keeps undocumented migrants healthy because they 'already have to bear all the weight of the adventure'. Her 'adventure' should therefore not be misunderstood as a purely hedonistic undertaking. The 'weight' is always present and, as with Suzanne, causes problems both physically and mentally:

So if one has […] a headache, it's perhaps because from time to time one is in a state of depression when thinking about the family. […] Because I spent the whole night thinking, thinking about my people, thinking about my family.

Again, similarly to Suzanne, Béatrice gets to know about the NGO early when she arrives in Switzerland, through the local diaspora. The community also provides her with housing and some child-minding jobs. As she says:

Some people already know how to get things done, as we are in an irregular situation, and also we don't have any work so we can't take out any health insurance. So, this way we are informed.

Béatrice is registered at the NGO with her name and date of birth. A short while later, she has a toothache that becomes so painful she needs treatment:

I needed to be given care immediately. Because there were already infections.

She decides to call Julia, the head of the NGO. Béatrice then describes in great detail, with precise reference to the specific days and hours, how Julia organizes a same-day after-hours dental appointment, accompanies her there because she does not know the city yet, and provides translation. Julia then sets up an urgent appointment for Béatrice with a surgeon at the dental surgery at seven o'clock the next morning. For Béatrice this non-bureaucratic and speedy treatment is a core moment of inclusion. This is confirmed at the end of the interview when, asked what she would like to add, she says:

That in Switzerland, at the NGO there are wonderful people who don't defer until tomorrow the things they can do today. Because it was an emergency. So, they always find a solution when facing an emergency.

This moment is the beginning of a lengthier period of treatment for Béatrice in the NGO's dentistry network, this moment of inclusion thus securing her stable dental care. As she explains, the surgeon, showing professional interest, found out that she has a tendency to lose teeth easily. There also seemed to be some teeth that had grown in the wrong direction, due to a specific morphology of her jaw. After having several teeth removed by the surgeon and consequently losing her ability to chew food, she needs an implant. Julia, having obtained the x-rays showing the state of her jaw after surgery, organizes a series of appointments with another dentist recommended by the surgeon. Asked more closely about these appointments, Béatrice says they were all set up by Julia. However, she stresses having gone there 'on my own and they would tell her [Julia] what had been done'. Again, Béatrice emphasises the importance of the professional's interest:

> *In the beginning* [...] *it was a bit difficult. Because when she saw the state of my mouth* [...] *'Why is it like this? What can we do?' But because she was good at her job, she found a solution. And for her, it was also a challenge.*

The dentist's view of Béatrice›s morphology as a challenge and an opportunity to stretch her professional practice plays an important part in Béatrice's lasting inclusion in healthcare, in Béatrice's view. She reports that the shape of her face changed during treatment and she had some issues accepting it, but states that she is very happy with it now. She still visits the dentist who did the implants for check-ups.

One question that comes to mind is why Béatrice never considered attending an emergency unit despite having such urgent problems with her teeth. Her response:

> *Well, the first thing they ask for is your identity card and you don't have any documents on you.*

According to the hospital staff, Béatrice's fear of being asked for an identity document is groundless. Andrew, the administrative employee, says: 'We couldn't care less about the legal status'. The doctor, Carl, agrees:

> *I don't really get told about it* [whether a patient is an undocumented migrant]. *Most of all, I don't know* [...] *what an undocumented migrant looks like, right?* [...] *We are not trained for that, and* [...] *I mean, it wouldn't change anything.*

Still, the fear of being exposed and subsequently deported when attending emergency care becomes clear when Béatrice tells of an acquaintance who had an ectopic pregnancy. The undocumented migrants whom she knew brought her to a hospital at the last minute, when she was already having convulsions and her limbs were going cold. They did not call an ambulance. Before driving, they called an

NGO and asked what they could do. Béatrice knows that no one who needs emergency care will be left to die and that, in life-threatening circumstances, care will be given first before payment is considered. Still, she assumes that inquiries about identity will be made:

> *They will first take care of you before asking you where you are from, what's your country of origin.*

But, and this is the other side of her story, Béatrice is amazed at how well her acquaintance was taken care of:

> *If you consider our hospitals, many would already be dead, but in Switzerland, people […] give their time for others. And, if I may say so, almost for free. For free. That's a great thing. It's great. Because* [at home] *for everything that is done you need to offer an incentive. But that's not the case here.*

Béatrice compares and contrasts her country of origin with Switzerland and highlights that, in Switzerland, delivery of care is independent of financial exchange or bribery. As we progress, we will encounter other examples of patients who value the predictability of a system free of corruption.

With this in mind, it must be said that Béatrice is right when she says that the care in such an urgent case is 'almost' for free. David, the general practitioner volunteering at the NGO, says:

> *Even when we send someone to an emergency department, they immediately check: is he able to pay?*

Indeed, as Andrew confirms, if they can talk to a patient before care is given and the administration becomes aware that costs are not covered by insurance, staff try to obtain a deposit of CHF 500. If this is not possible, care is given anyway, as Andrew explains:

> *We do inform the doctor that the patient can't pay the deposit. And then the doctor simply takes the history, carries out diagnosis and provides treatment. But he also assesses, well, whether things can be postponed until the finances are sorted. Or whether we have to* [do something immediately], *in which case we do it.*

If patients provide an address, however, they are pursued for payment. An undocumented migrant would therefore either have to pay for the care, give a false address, or deal with being pursued, risking exposure once again. Andrew explains that the hospital's canton does not refund costs for the treatments of patients without insurance.

If a patient admits to not having insurance but lives in the hospital's canton, the administrative staff will make them sign a form that is sent to the canton's officials who are responsible for mandatory social insurances, such as health insurance. These officials will then enroll the patient in an insurance scheme. The patient on the other hand, then has to pay the monthly premium However, the head of the NGO knows that in these situations, undocumented migrants will sometimes give the wrong address, resulting in a futile administrative process.

Returning then to the NGO, we have seen that it plays a key role in migrants' ongoing inclusion in healthcare. To some extent this role continues throughout the entire process, with Julia receiving medical reports and organizing all the appointments. Migrants therefore depend on the NGO and its network of volunteers for healthcare even after their transformative moment of inclusion. The NGO, however, depends on its professionals, although it is difficult to find dentists willing to work extra hours and for reduced fees. Béatrice says that both of the dentists caring for her had previously worked in areas that were riven by civil war, and also in developing countries, and Julia adds that she has found it easier to motivate dentists to help if they are or have been migrants themselves. Again, personal engagement and goodwill is needed. The resulting lack of formal agreements and the high cost of treatment prompt the NGO to closely monitor professionals' interactions with patients, so that they can mediate quickly in case of difficulties. Undocumented migrants are sometime unreliable at keeping appointments, which can be a source of problems. As Julia says:

> *Especially with the dentists I'm really pedantic, I accompany almost every single person. Only when I see that people are really reliable [...], only then do I tell them they can go on their own.*

As the nurse, Melanie, says, at the NGO itself, flexibility is needed:

> *Overall, I had to learn to deal with that, people either attend or they don't. For whatever reasons, maybe they are working, or they forgot, or they couldn't afford the train fare. [...] You know, we're not like in a hospital, where you then go, well they didn't attend this time, we may as well not take them next time.*

*That's not how it is here. We say hey, we are here for these people and if they
don't attend, they will have their reasons.*

For instance, Béatrice says that she might not always be reachable, as,
when child-minding, she sometimes stays in another city for several
weeks and cannot leave during that time. Certainly, the professionals
in the NGO's network are not always willing or able to offer such
flexibility.

Until she is prompted, Béatrice doesn't address the financial aspect
of her treatment. Asked about her contribution to costs, she says she can
make it up with her little jobs and again mentions Julia as her first point
of contact for these issues.

The NGO has a fixed budget of CHF 500 per patient per year. The
primary strategy to counter this financial precarity is to require patients
to contribute towards the costs of their treatment. But there is no clear
procedure for the personnel of the NGO to assess a patient's financial
capacity. As Julia says:

I have to negotiate with them each time. And there is nothing I can refer to.

Julia describes how she has developed 'a feeling' for these things, and
attempts to 'take people at their word'. She wants them to understand
that 'everything is not for free'. In the case of dental care, patients
are asked to pay at least one quarter of the total costs in instalments.
Sometimes, money can also be reallocated from patients who have not
incurred high costs. Sometimes, patients defraud their way into care, as
Melanie explains:

*Well, I have also been tricked by some, in that I sent them to the dentist and they
never returned. [laughs] Yeah, of course, that money, I never saw it again.*

As we will see later on, for various reasons patients sometimes obtain
healthcare through fraud and lies. Such means are judged by society to
be morally wrong or even illegal, so these attempts at inclusion further
marginalize undocumented migrants.

Béatrice's story confirms what we heard in Suzanne's account:
inclusion in healthcare requires inclusion in a community and in a
system of paid work, in order to establish a good living situation and to
contribute towards the costs of care.

For Béatrice, inclusion in healthcare at the NGO and its network has very positive consequences, as it enables stable and lasting care for her dental problem. Furthermore, the unexpectedly quick and non-bureaucratic provision of appointments proved to be very important for Béatrice's lasting inclusion in a programme of treatment. More negative associations with healthcare are revealed when Béatrice is talking about emergency care. Here she conflates the idea of exclusion from healthcare with administrative exclusion due to her lack of legal status. Therefore, the condition of being 'undocumented' in itself excludes people from emergency care. Furthermore, the financial responsibilities of inclusion are also difficult to undertake and may put undocumented migrants at risk of deportation, should they be pursued for costs. Financial difficulties therefore increase the likelihood of patients being excluded from healthcare.

Listening to the two nurses working at the NGO, the reader can also start to see that such quick and non-bureaucratic aid and professional engagement stem from an ongoing effort by professionals. This involves the establishment of stable agreements, in a situation where goodwill, personal engagement and organizational flexibility are particularly necessary. In addition, financial insecurity, which brings with it the risk of exclusion from healthcare, is partly transferred from patients to the NGO, thus intensifying the organization's dependence on the goodwill of the individuals in its network.

The engagement and interest shown by the professionals whom she encountered were important conditions for inclusion for Béatrice. Such qualities would probably also be identified as significant by patients belonging to the wider population, demonstrating that inclusion in healthcare need not, in Béatrice's case, be determined solely by factors that relate to her legal status. Another important aspect of her inclusion is more specific to Béatrice's situation: the NGO's dependence on the professionals in its network requires a certain passivity from her. However, her statements show that she values the act of attending appointments on her own, so it is important for her to maintain a degree of autonomy whilst achieving inclusion.

Peter: 'These people are now like my family'

In 2016, 13,526 people were denied asylum or temporary admission in Switzerland, corresponding to 51% of all asylum claims (Staatssekretariat für Migration 2017:16). Some failed asylum seekers appeal to the administrative court, while others leave the country or go into hiding. Still others live on so called 'emergency assistance' organized by the state; despite this state support, they are undocumented migrants insofar as they have no right to stay in the country. If not housed by friends, they live in emergency accommodation where they also receive food. Some of them are given about CHF 60 a week, others are handed vouchers. Failed asylum seekers do have access to a health insurance policy, provided by a special scheme, which is also given to asylum seekers while the assessment process is still underway. Healthcare can then be accessed via the asylum centre's staff and is covered by the insurance. Failed asylum seekers sometimes live in this situation for years and are under the constant threat of being deported.

Peter, a man in his thirties, is one of these failed asylum seekers. In addition to the rejection of his application for asylum, his identity documents were confiscated during the assessment process. He consequently has no documents at all relating to his identity.

At the start of the interview, he explains that he left his country after having been tortured during an eight-month imprisonment. His journey to Switzerland included a difficult stay of several months in Greece, from where he finally, with some additional financial help from his family, reached Switzerland in a truck. Arriving in an asylum camp about mid-2011, he told the staff there that

> *I have health problems. When I* [was] *in* [my home country] *they* […] *tortured me too much.* […] *And sometimes I feel very bad. I* […] *think that maybe tomorrow I'll die.*

After he was moved to a transit centre and thereafter to a cantonal centre, he again told staff about his health issues, but he was still not given any care in this respect. During this time, Peter also had difficult experiences with a general practitioner:

> [I said] *'I have a problem'. He asked 'why do you come here so often?'* [I came]
> *two or three times during one week because* [...] *my health was very bad. When*
> *I go* [again he asked] *'why are you here?' I say 'you don't know anything'.*

The same doctor diagnosed Peter with a stomach problem and subsequently sent him for surgery at a hospital. But apparently he did not recognize, or could not adequately respond to, Peter's mental health problems. Peter's inclusion in healthcare remained partial.

Again, his interactions with healthcare staff in the hospital and the surgery itself were good experiences, and Peter reports having been well informed and treated. During the interview, he explains in detail how the endoscopy was explained to him. He reports feeling afraid:

> *You know, in my land, sometimes some people who are having an endoscopy,*
> [...] *they have much pain* [...] *and then they say, 'ah you may change completely*
> [...] *it's not good'.*

Laughing, he says that after the surgery,

> *when I woke up, they said 'ok it's finished'. I thought that maybe they start now.*
> *They say 'it's finished'. I say 'What? Ah, it's finished'.*

Still, his mental health problems remained untreated as his application for asylum was rejected and he was transferred once again. For Peter, every transfer meant an unannounced and unexpected disruption that was difficult to understand. Throughout the interview it was not easy to follow with precision all of the different places he was transferred to. The hospital's doctor, Carl, confirms that this is also a difficulty for healthcare professionals: 'In Switzerland you don't know how the patient did at his last placement'. At his next placement, in emergency accommodation, Peter's mental health problems are still not adequately treated:

> *They gave us too much medicine. 'You use this one, this is very good, you use*
> *this one this is very good'.* [...] *But I think* [...] *I have another problem. And*
> *they gave me another medicine, because 'ah, we have a sample here'.*

Adding to his difficulties, there is the insecurity associated with life as an undocumented migrant, at the constant mercy of the authorities. This is well illustrated by Peter's account of an encounter with police at a time when he was already receiving treatment in the NGO's network:

We [Peter and a friend] *were in a car and police came and they* [stopped] *us and they said: 'What is this?', and I say: 'No no no' and then they caught me and one night I was* [in prison]. *I told them that I* [...] *have a doctor. They say no. The next day a translator came and they say: 'Why you are not going back to your country?' I say that I have problems there. They said: 'It's better for you to go back'. The next day, another of these guys came with me to a big police station.* [...] *They took my fingerprints again and then they said: 'Now you are released'. And every time, when you see the police you are afraid. If they catch you or if they* [stop] *you then you have problems again.*

As the police do not take Peter's reference to his treatment within the NGO's network into consideration, he is left with no other option than to try and explain why he does not want to go back to his home country. He is therefore reduced once more to his status as failed asylum seeker, once again having to undergo the typical steps of the asylum procedure, such as providing his fingerprints. The way Peter relates this episode shows how helpless he feels during the interaction with police. He concludes:

You know I left [my country] *to feel safe* [...] *but here it's the same situation. Every time I'm afraid* [...] *when police* [stop] *me.*

Peter is put in touch with the NGO at the beginning of 2013, one and a half years after his arrival in Switzerland, via a counselling service for undocumented migrants:

First, when I was here, when I slept, I saw everything that happened to me in my land. And I could not sleep well and I could not eat and everything was very bad, and then I came here and then they gave me treatment and slowly, slowly I am feeling better.

Inclusion at the NGO is a turning point for Peter twice over. First, he is referred from the NGO to outpatient psychiatric care. This therapy, he says, is doing him a lot of good. Again, he stresses the importance of continuity of treatment:

Because, [the psychiatrist] *knows me very well* [...] *and he knows my situation he treated me very slowly, slowly.*

Peter's 'slowly, slowly' marks a contrast to the haste and disruption he describes in his life as a failed asylum seeker. In addition, the NGO is an important place to help him address some of the problems his legal status is causing him. Echoing Suzanne and Béatrice, he talks about the difficulties he experiences because he is unable to help his family. He becomes very sad at this point of the interview, but at the same time he relates how the NGO addresses this issue:

> *I cannot do anything for my family. [...] And I am very thankful to [Julia] because [...] she asked me: 'Why are you worried?' I said 'my mother is very sick'. And she said 'ok don't worry. You bring me all the reports'. [...] And she looked at it and also discussed it with doctors and she gave me medicine I'm sending to my mother.*

In this instance, the NGO gives Peter the ability to act upon a health issue he would not otherwise be able to address. A bit later, he says about the NGO:

> *You know now these people are like my family. Because, I don't have another family. But I've spent a long time with these guys and [...] when I have any problem, then I discuss [it] with these people and sometimes I feel happiness and I discuss it with these guys.*

We can see here that for Peter, the role of the NGO and the meaning of inclusion in healthcare are quite broad. The NGO's professionals are described as a family, essential to Peter's health and wellbeing. This statement at once expresses the immense benefit that both the NGO and psychiatric treatment have provided but also the loss of social ties and securities that Peter has experienced. This account also shows that, for Peter, inclusion in healthcare cannot be seen as tied to one locality or person. His health is embedded in a wider context, encompassing family left behind and new connections built up in the context of immigration.

For the NGO's professionals, these challenging situations are a vital part of their motivation. Julia emphasises her interest in transcultural care and sees her work as being at the nexus between culture and health. For her, this means identifying a patient's needs and his or her way of communicating them. This begins with listening to patients:

> *it's almost as if you use* [their concrete health problem] *as a stepping stone to gently approach the much more complicated problem, that of their legal status.*

Melanie, the nurse, again contrasts the NGO with ordinary care organizations:

It's not at all like care as you know it from a hospital, or an old age home, or home care services. [...] They come here with everything and they bring along the most complex stories. Not all of them, but things become quite complex very quickly when their health is impaired in some way.

A further important quality of inclusion as far as the professionals are concerned is to build up trust with the patients. As David states: 'Even as an NGO, you don't just have their trust'. Melanie echoes this sentiment:

When I work as a nurse in hospital, and I enter the room in my white uniform, people [...] assume my good intentions. Here, it's not like that.

This again essentially means that there is a need to take time to get to know patients better, as she describes:

I think our advantage here is that we can take our time in most cases, or we invite someone to come in a second time. And I think for our patients that's extremely important. They feel taken seriously, they feel respected.

Certainly, the biggest issue that still affects Peter's health is the threat caused by his immigration status, which excludes him from most parts of civil life. Living for much of the time at a friend's place, he remains uncertain that he won't be transferred again, or even deported. His inclusion in healthcare thus remains precarious, while he has developed some problems with his blood pressure and heart. For instance, at the last centre where he stayed, he could go to a general practitioner who 'treated me very well and regularly and also he's very nice, a very, very nice guy'. But after his most recent transfer, he doesn't know, yet again, which doctor he is allowed to visit.

Peter's story shows the difficulties that undocumented migrants can have when it comes to inclusion in healthcare for certain conditions, even if they are insured. Accessing the NGO is the most important moment for inclusion, not only because it leads, finally, to addressing Peter's condition through adequate therapy, but also because it provides an opportunity to talk about the problems that stem directly from his legal status. We have seen with Béatrice's story that the administrative aspects of inclusion sometimes have to be adapted to the specific circumstances of undocumented migrants. With Peter's story, we begin to see that in some cases the care process itself has to take specific needs into account. Peter needs to talk about his lack of perspective, fear of deportation, or issues such as caring for a family left behind. This in turn enables the patient to confront health issues and to take an active part in his own care.

On the other hand, for specific physical conditions and the treatments they require, inclusion in healthcare can be quite unproblematic and the interaction between medical personnel and patient does not require special measures. In this respect Peter's statement echoes the stories of Suzanne and Béatrice.

Importantly though, Peter's account shows how difficult it can be to provide continuous inclusion both during and after the asylum assessment process. Being moved from one centre to the next not only contributes to the insecurity of the patients, but also cuts existing ties to healthcare professionals who consequently cannot get to know their patients and, instead of coming to recognize more hidden health issues as a result of increased patient familiarity, end up being overstretched themselves, adding to patient exclusion from healthcare.

Maria: 'I was in bondage but I didn't know'

At the NGO, about 90% of the patients do not have health insurance. As already discussed in the last chapter, for the general population of undocumented migrants in Switzerland, this percentage is estimated to be close to 80%-90%. It is unknown how many undocumented migrants have conditions that require medical treatment, though, given these numbers, features of the case we are about to discuss might well be common to at least some of them. Other patients without insurance who manage to access the NGO and get treatment through its networks might also share Maria's experiences.

Maria, a woman in her late thirties, fled political upheavals in her country of origin. She was imprisoned and gave birth to her son during migration. Arriving in Switzerland in 1997, she was treated in a psychiatric hospital for about two or three years. Though her memory of the time has become blurry, she does her best to explain her condition:

> *It was like I was dying. There was no life in me, I just knew that I was still living. For years [...] I had a stiff neck.*

Upon her release from the hospital sometime between 1999 and 2000, her request for asylum was turned down. But because she had just married a man with a Swiss residency permit, she was allowed to stay. Her son was naturalized. However, because she and her son were ill-treated by her husband, she decided to get a divorce even though that meant losing her right to remain in Switzerland. As she did not dare work on the black market, she also lost her health insurance.

Some time passed and she became engaged to a new partner around 2008. But this marriage is not recognized by the authorities. The procedures to legalize her stay are still ongoing, and have, in her view, taken on Kafkaesque dimensions:

> *I had to appeal to the state. The state refused. Then my lawyer said there's another option, it's called federal* [court]. *Then they refuse.* [...] *So, I appealed to the* [state secretary for] *immigration, the state* [court] *and the federal* [court] *three times. So I do the appeal nine times. So it cost my husband more than 20,000 Swiss Francs.*

She reports that the immigration authorities tried to deport her several times but could not execute the deportation order. She describes the fear this has caused her:

> *If they want to deport you, they will come to your house early in the morning. So then after they attempted and they couldn't succeed, I became afraid. Even in the night* [...] *if I should hear a car, I would get out of bed to go and see if it's the police.* [...] *So it was really a terrible experience.*

She highlights another important aspect of her situation, which also impacts other undocumented migrants' health, as we will see later:

> *I'm ashamed to tell people my story.* [...] *Because people sometimes they will laugh at you when you tell them you have a problem. I always keep everything inside, keep everything inside.*

Finally, she directly connects some of her health problems to her legal status: 'I develop [problems with my] blood pressure because of this paper problem'. But the situation is such that she cannot address these issues. She understands that with all the money her husband is putting into the legal process, he cannot afford health insurance for her on top of that.

With her legal situation remaining unresolved, Maria's health goes from bad to worse during a period of seven years from 2005 onwards: 'So my blood pressure was high, I was sick, you know it started slowly

slowly'. A whole cluster of symptoms built up in severity during this time:

> *That tiredness. […] I cannot describe it. […] if I should raise my hand […] it's a
> big job for me. My heart is beating fast* [because of a] *small thing. I don't enjoy
> anything, I don't enjoy my body, I don't enjoy anything. Just to sleep and cover
> myself. Two weeks before my menstruation, I'm in another world. Two weeks
> after my menstruation is like war for me. I cannot even describe the pain. The
> pain is even more than punishment.*

She knows there is medication that would help address her blood pressure, but it requires a prescription. Fraud becomes seemingly her only option:

> *Sometimes I just have to go and lie to the pharmacy because I don't have
> insurance.* [I say] *that I want to send this to […] my mom.*

In this way, Maria sometimes obtains medication to treat her high blood pressure. At other times she is not so lucky and is only given herbal remedies. Later in the interview, she explains how her success at obtaining effective medication is dependent upon the pharmacy's staff:

> *Because they used to have different people at the pharmacy. So there's a man*
> [who] *would always sell it to me. But if it's just this lady, she will tell me 'ah
> no'.*

Again, the patient must depend on goodwill, but also on the professional's willingness to bend the rules. Her attempts at inclusion therefore marginalize her and also impose a potential risk on the professional involved. To treat her many other problems, Maria's only option is Dafalgan, a brand of paracetamol: 'I'm taking Dafalgan like fruit'.

Maria contacted the NGO in 2012 through the same organization as Peter. From there, she was first referred to be examined at a lab and by a gynaecologist in the network. At both places, but especially at the gynaecologist, Maria reports that she received very good and humane treatment. 'I even didn't have to pay'. Again, the fact that there was no immediate need to pay in order to receive care is surprising and contributes to a positive experience. Maria is diagnosed with a fibroid in her breast and uterus, the latter causing heavy menstruation. She is also diagnosed with iron deficiency anaemia, high blood pressure, and depression.

She is given a prescription for blood pressure medicine at the NGO, her low iron is treated at the lab, and her depression is also addressed. As a result, after over seven years, she regains an awareness of the difference between good and bad health. It is her most important moment of inclusion in healthcare:

> *You know after a while you don't know what's normal and what's not normal. Yeah. You see before, when I woke up with this headache, after some time, my body was like ah, it's normal life, to get up with a headache. But like three months after the treatment I started to feel good in my body. Then I started to say 'oh God, so this is how I am supposed to live'. So it is like, before I was in bondage but I didn't know. I knew but I didn't really know that I can be free. So I didn't know that this suffering could be avoided. I thought ah, that is how I will live. That is how it is. But the day that I started to get better, it's like my eyes opened and I'm in another world.*

At one point, Maria addresses the recorder directly, as if willing it to pass a message to an audience:

> *I thank* [the NGO] *one million times.* [...] *Because maybe I could have been a stroke patient.* [...] *I appreciate their good work. If God blesses me in life and gives me a job I will join to support them. They see illegal people as human beings.*

Maria's statement honours the work of the NGO and echoes Peter's sentiments, but, at the same time, it highlights Maria's dependence on the charitable organization.

Importantly, the fibroid causing her heavy menstruation requires surgical intervention. Unfortunately, such a procedure is impossible to finance without insurance. Maria is resigned:

> *It will take a miracle.* [...] *But I just pray that the immigration* [office] *should answer me. Quick. So that I can get a job.*

Thus, even though Maria has been freed from the 'bondage' she did not know she was suffering, she is still far from freedom. The fibroid, but also her difficulties concerning her legal status, have now been weighing on her for a very long time.

Theoretically, she and her partner could choose to cease their legal efforts and use the money to pay for insurance instead, but that would terminate any hope of regularizing her legal status, of living a life without fear, and of gaining legal employment. As Julia puts it, 'we are all born with this insurance'. Indeed, Swiss citizens are included into healthcare from birth by virtue of their citizenship and later thanks to their employment which allows them to pay for their insurance policy. Furthermore, if Swiss residents cannot afford health insurance, they can rely on social welfare. In Maria's case however we are for the first time confronted with a situation in which the lack of work and the absence of citizenship directly prevent a patient from undergoing treatment, something that goes against the common perception that in Switzerland healthcare is within everybody's reach.

As in the case of Béatrice, professionals work under constant financial pressure in the background to provide even the partial and precarious inclusion afforded to undocumented migrants. To send uninsured patients for additional care outside the NGO is, according to David,

> *always problematic. Well, I should say, almost always. […] It's immediately a question of money. […] In my surgery I was used to being generous, like [for example] everything that was a potential diagnosis was checked in the lab. Here, we can't do that. So I have to restrict myself to what is really important to know. […] It's a constant balancing act. How much risk can we shoulder ourselves, and when has the line been reached where […] a more detailed examination or a specialist or the like is indispensable.*

Maria adds to the doctor's statement when she recounts her first visit to the lab:

> *I think at the lab they made a mistake. […] The doctor here said I should do like two or three tests. So they did like ten tests for me [laughs] by mistake. So […] they find out that I have anaemia.*

For Maria, this was a lucky accident. For the NGO though, such mistakes can rapidly turn into financial problems, as David explains:

> *A young woman had a broken finger, and I wasn't sure whether it was broken or just badly bruised. So I sent her to [a hospital] with a referral for an x-ray. But there, she was seen by an orthopaedic surgeon, who then immediately operated on her. From a medical perspective, perfect. But in terms of cost, something like six or seven thousand Swiss francs. And then, afterwards, the discussion: 'Hey, we'd only asked for an x-ray'. That got very complicated.*

The NGO's close monitoring of the interactions between its patients and the healthcare professionals in its network, which we encountered in Béatrice's story, is undertaken partly in order to avoid situations like these.

Again, for the professionals of the NGO, the patients' financial difficulties are mirrored by their own restrictions. Asked about how well they think the Swiss healthcare system functions with regard to care for undocumented migrants, David says: 'What seems very problematic to me, is how much of it is tied to money'. Melanie wonders why most healthcare for undocumented migrants is provided by NGOs. For her, it would be best to

incorporate this into a regular structure as with other things in a canton. Because then we would have funding and also some structures.

In Béatrice and Suzanne's accounts, settling in helped with their inclusion into healthcare. Maria's story illustrates just how difficult acquiring insurance and healthcare can be when the person involved has no income because she has no access to either the legal or the illegal labor market. In order to keep a very small amount of control over one's healthcare and health, engaging in fraud while depending upon someone's complicity is an option. Marginalization is the consequence. Another aspect of the situation is that a sense of what it feels like to be healthy is lost over time. This is clearly demonstrated by the contrast Maria describes between her state before and after her inclusion at the NGO and in its network.

If we combine these accounts with Peter's story, we are building a clearer sense of the mental pressures that weigh on undocumented migrants living at the mercy of the immigration authorities. At the same time, we see the importance of inclusion in addressing these specific issues and giving the patient room to talk about what otherwise must remain in shadow. We also see once more the extent to which the undocumented migrants are dependent on the NGO for inclusion in healthcare, and overall we have a clearer picture of how financial restrictions and dependence on the goodwill of others are common to both patients and the NGO.

Finally, a further interesting aspect of Maria's story is the paradoxical 'choice' by which aiming for inclusion in healthcare involves taking actions that could harm one's health. Inclusion in an official economy, a job market, and a system of social welfare are unspoken prerequisites for inclusion in healthcare. As these are lacking, Maria's only feasible strategies for inclusion worsen her health at the same time. If she decides to take out insurance, she has to give up her efforts to legalize her stay. This worsens her health by completely eliminating the hope that she will ever escape her situation of being undocumented. Conversely, if Maria decides to continue her efforts to legalize her stay, she worsens her health by leaving her fibroid untreated. Maria's will not be the only case that results in this unpalatable choice. To a certain extent, such paradoxical consequences might also exist for citizens in precarious financial situations, but they appear here with a force and brutality hardly imaginable for people who, in the end, can still rely upon social welfare.

Jonathan: 'I had no place to go'

The Swiss law on asylum states that 'asylum seekers must state any serious health problems of relevance' (AsylG Art. 26 al. 1) during the asylum process. Usually, requests for asylum on purely medical grounds are quickly turned down. However, in some cases asylum seekers are granted a residency of one year with a permit, because in the country they have left behind

> a necessary treatment is not granted or not granted sufficiently and the return would result in a rapid and life-threatening deterioration of health. (Der Schweizerische Bundesrat 2016)[1]

In 2015, 201 people were granted a temporary residency exclusively for health reasons. This amounts to 4% of the one-year permits granted that year (Der Schweizerische Bundesrat 2016).

It is 2016 and Jonathan has been granted a one-year permit for medical reasons only weeks before his interview with me takes place. Had the interview happened later, he would probably have cited this as

---

1   'wenn eine notwendige Behandlung im Heimat- oder Herkunftsstaat gar nicht oder nicht ausreichend zur Verfügung steht und die Rückkehr zu einer raschen und lebensgefährdenden Beeinträchtigung des Gesundheitszustandes führt'.

his most important moment of inclusion in healthcare. But as the event is so recent, and he has already been in Switzerland for eight years, Jonathan concentrates on the time before the permit was granted.

Jonathan's story starts with the deaths of his two brothers; like him, both suffered from a mixed form of type I and type II diabetes. His sister advised him to leave his home country and the family started selling its cows so that Jonathan could afford a safe trip to Switzerland in 2008. However, on his journey he had no means to care for his diabetes. At the time of his arrival in Switzerland, he was immediately hospitalized:

> *The doctor checked my sugar and it was, oh, very, very, very serious. So, immediately they took me to the hospital. I stayed there maybe one or two weeks […] because the diabetes was very, oh, no insulin […] you know.*

From this time onwards, Jonathan enrolled in the asylum process. His request was rejected by the authorities because — according to the officials — diabetes can be treated in Jonathan's home country. In 2010 Jonathan decided to go into hiding. Other than Béatrice, Maria and Suzanne, he did not have any contacts in Switzerland. Trying to get work, especially while suffering from untreated diabetes, did not even seem to be worth considering, so Jonathan adopted strategies to take care of his health that harmed him further:

> *I eat everything, which is not allowed you know. But I don't have no choice.*

With no access to insulin, he took up walking in an attempt, as he says, 'to get the sugar down' and states that this caused a lesion on his foot that did not heal. For Jonathan, this wound presented a severe physical problem, and, in light of the circumstances of his brothers' deaths, was also a source of a very profound fear for his life:

> *The foot was also a very big problem for me because my brother had it in my country and he couldn't make it.*

After some months, Jonathan's next attempt to be included in healthcare was to file for asylum a second time:

> *It was very, very difficult for me; I didn't have medicaments, so I was sick. So people advised me: 'You have to make another asylum* [claim] *because you are sick'. And this was very dangerous.*

We will see later, when discussing Fanny's story, that in certain very serious and urgent circumstances, undocumented migrants may engage in the asylum process for purely medical reasons, which also means facing an increased risk of deportation. Jonathan, however, did not see any other possibility to handle his rapidly worsening diabetes and he says that he was again sent to hospital immediately. At the end of the treatment he reports that he was discharged with 'a lot of medicine'.

During the previous and the subsequent stage, the conditions for Jonathan in Switzerland were similar to those in his home country. He finds it very hard to understand why, in a country with such a good healthcare system, he was not given care during these periods:

> *It was even a surprise for me, you know. I said wow, I am here but I have no help. Yeah, I always think about this, you know. I said, never mind the paper; I am a human being. The paper they can forget about it, but for my life, you know. […] I was thinking that maybe if I came here, it would be better. But […] [it was] not like that, ah. Not like that.*

Finally, some months later in 2011, an acquaintance told him about the NGO. When Jonathan attended for the first time, he travelled there by public transport without a valid ticket and risked being caught by the conductor and thus discovered. Given Jonathan's state at that moment in time, it is easily understandable that the care provided at the NGO and through its network was a turning point in his story:

> *This means that if I don't […] see these people so quickly, then it would have been too late.*

Like Peter, he describes a slow process of building relationships, of getting to know and trust others: 'We started, you know, not very quickly, but slowly, slowly, knowing each other'. This process resulted in decisive moments that shaped Jonathan's inclusion in healthcare. Given his very precarious social situation, the NGO made an exception and financed his insurance itself and therefore, for Jonathan, the insurance itself was a less decisive or visible factor, and he only mentions it at the very end of the interview.

Much more important for him is the fact that he is taken care of by a diabetes counsellor within the NGO's network. She became an important person for Jonathan, opening up other possibilities for inclusion, and thus substantially contributing to his health.

But inclusion is still sometimes difficult. For instance, due to medical complications, Jonathan sometimes needs to access emergency services. One night, when he was still homeless, he had a very bad stomach ache:

> *So I don't know what to do* [...] *I have no money to call the taxi. I don't* [...] *contact the ambulance because if* [...] *I contact the ambulance what can I do? I have no papers, I have no insurance card, nothing. So, I said, these people in the hospital know me* [...] *I have to go by myself. So that night I walk to the hospital from* [a place about one hour away on foot]. [...] *I have to walk tall* [holding himself upright], *because of the police. When I walk I have to sit, I walk, I sit, oh,* [...] *that day I was thinking that I'm going to die.*

The lack of a document to show to the ambulance drivers is here contrasted with the advantage of knowing people in the hospital. This emphasises again the importance of, and dependence on, personal relationships when it comes to inclusion in healthcare. The emergency unit itself will take care of him as he has insurance, something that at this point in time Jonathan has no doubt about. But because he lacks an insurance card he walks for an hour to the next hospital, late at night and in a critical state of health. Fear of being stopped by the police accompanies him all the way.

In a non life-threatening situation if a patient does not have an insurance card, this can raise professionals' suspicions about coverage of costs and thus foster exclusion. Jonathan reports that he had to remind doctors that they would be paid to treat him, as, despite being an undocumented migrant, he did have insurance. Only the reference to the NGO made them 'relax' according to Jonathan. As he saw it, he had to handle the professionals' fear of unpaid costs, even though he was the one in need of help and support. He contrasts this with the situation at the NGO where 'people [...] don't care if I have paper or not'. As the diabetes counsellor, Caroline, says about Jonathan:

> *He has always received treatment because he had insurance, and then it depended a bit on the individual people.*

She states that sometimes there were 'reservations' or language problems, but on other occasions people took extra care because they knew the patient was an undocumented migrant.

Certainly, receiving care and being able to obtain it on his own at times was a big step forward for Jonathan. Still, bringing us back to his social situation, he says of the NGO:

> *I give them a tough time you know. Because* [laughing] *I have no choice you know. When I knock the door and this lady opened the door and saw me she said 'oh my God* [laughing] *it's him again'. Yeah, because she knew that at the moment I get inside I just start to complain. You know, I was a headache. I had no place to go, no place to go.*

With regard to the social situation of undocumented migrants, Jonathan presents a paradigmatic case of what happens when inclusion in healthcare remains very haphazard due to a combination of multiple exclusions.

We can elaborate upon this point by returning to the professionals' point of view. Jonathan's diabetes counsellor, Caroline, says that with the insurance, she was able to prescribe insulin, needles, and syringes for him, 'just like for a Swiss patient'. But it was difficult for the homeless Jonathan to store the insulin. He says that he sometimes kept it in a little stream where he could cool it. Sometimes he also stored the insulin with some colleagues who lived in a nearby centre for asylum seekers. He is proud that he found ways to help himself even in difficult situations. But in the end, the insulin 'didn't help him much because he had nothing to eat', as Caroline explains. She also reports that she has not been able to properly adjust Jonathan's medication because he was always afraid he might become hypoglycaemic in public and then be found out by the police.

Caroline reports that she and a doctor at her hospital did a lot of 'social work' to improve Jonathan's situation. She mentions the following activities: organizing housing, organizing money for podiatry, accompanying Jonathan to show him the place where he could obtain orthopaedic shoes, forwarding bills to the NGO, giving financial guarantees, acting as a contact person for other hospitals and informing them about Jonathan's health status and medication, informing Jonathan about appointments, organizing surgery for his foot and eyes, and providing Jonathan with her private phone number. However, even Caroline's resources are not limitless. For instance, when her colleagues from the hospital call her to inform her that Jonathan has nowhere to go after he wakes up from anaesthesia, she cannot help either. Together with the hospital doctor and the head of the NGO, Caroline always tried to find a way to maintain 'a small pot of petty cash' reserved to help Jonathan. She concludes:

We can do an amazing job. [...] Yet, I've never gone home with a clear conscience because you just know everything else doesn't work, and then the best healthcare is useless.

For the professionals, this creates a paradoxical situation, as Caroline explains:

Sometimes we were almost happy when he had another episode. Then he could go back to hospital for three or four days, and he had something to eat, a shower, a warm bed.

Carl, who is a doctor in the emergency unit of a hospital, confirms this by saying that patients sometimes attend the unit in the winter because they have no place to sleep:

I don't think our hospital is set up for this. [...] There are no real [associated] social services as there are in other countries.

The asylum process enabled Jonathan to access healthcare at the beginning of his story, and now healthcare organizations help him to obtain some minimal social inclusion. This in turn makes healthcare interventions more effective.

Jonathan's social situation and his ability to look after his own health and healthcare improved only when he was granted a one-year permit. NGO employees and healthcare professionals helped him to file the application this time. It was accepted because the immigration authorities recognized that, unlike the diabetes itself, the long-term effects of Jonathan's illness cannot be treated in his home country. It was thus the restricted nature of Jonathan's inclusion in healthcare in Switzerland, particularly during the early stages of his time in the country, that finally ensured the success of the application for the temporary permit. Exclusion from healthcare therefore made possible Jonathan's political inclusion, and thus his ultimate inclusion in healthcare beyond the charitable support of the NGO.

Given his very precarious social situation, it is not surprising that Jonathan does not spend a lot of time thinking about how his insurance is organized and paid for. Still, in the background, numerous institutional and organizational arrangements between the NGO and insurance companies have to be made in order to insure undocumented migrants.

In Jonathan's case, the NGO first provides an address for all correspondence with the insurance company. The NGO also finds a person with a Swiss residency permit in order for the relevant financial transactions to take place via a Swiss bank account. However, the insurance company also has to make special arrangements. Patricia's employers have created a special department that deals exclusively with asylum seekers and undocumented migrants. As Patricia explains, the employees in this department

> *deal with the more delicate cases [...] and nobody else does, because only very few have that level of training.*

The training and sensitivity is mainly required for the process of verifying that the applicant indeed has his or her residency in the country. Insurance employees must not contact the municipality for this verification. Furthermore, it is important that the staff of the insurance company know how to react to inquiries by municipalities, as Patricia points out:

> *When someone calls from the municipality and makes enquiries about somebody, then we ask them why they're calling and we tell them that we're not permitted to give any information. In those moments, we're very unapologetic and very unrelenting because they're just determined to get their hands on this data by all means necessary.*

Once all the prerequisites have been arranged by the NGO and the insurance company, Patricia explains that the application for insurance has to be filed in a rather unusual way:

> *[A regular application]* is seen by umpteen people, from the scanning centre to the internal mail clerk, everybody can look at it because the document is open. And later we also scan it into the system, electronically. And we aim to avoid all of that by saying that [you have to send it directly] to our department [using] a code number indicating that it's about an undocumented migrant. With those [NGOs] that we have [this] agreement with, that works. And also, [using this system] no applications are lost. [You see], that is the risk when someone just applies [by themselves], there's a real risk that the application ends up just anywhere.

Not all insurers are trusted by the NGO to guarantee this level of data protection and exactitude. Once more, undocumented migrants are included in healthcare thanks to specific arrangements and personal contacts that build a relationship of trust, this time between organizations. The personal investment and understanding of the insurance employees is also needed, as Patricia describes:

> *What I personally think is very important is the personal* [attitude] *and awareness that these people really have nothing here, they didn't choose this situation.*

From a patient's perspective, all these special arrangements and the need to use someone else's address and bank account details make them heavily dependent on others for their inclusion in healthcare.

Finally, we must explain why Jonathan has no insurance card. This is quite a common problem for undocumented migrants. We have already encountered it in the story about Nicolas' hospital visit in Chapter One. In order to issue an insurance card to an undocumented migrant, the insurance company has to put in a request for an 'Alters und Hinterlassenenversicherung' (AHV) number, the Swiss social security number. This procedure is required for foreign diplomatic staff, for example. But as Patricia states:

> *Insurers tend to be reluctant to issue* [insurance] *cards, especially for undocumented migrants, because one doesn't know what they want to use it for, are they going to get medicine and so on. That said, I must say our insurance is not like that.*

The suspicion that the card will be misused is the difference between the case of diplomatic dignitaries and that of undocumented migrants, and as a result insurers do not issue cards to undocumented migrants, or do so very unwillingly. For the patients though, the card may be very important in order to be included in healthcare. From the perspective of the administrative staff of the organizations that deliver healthcare, the absence of the card can create suspicion about the availability of financial coverage, as Patricia explains:

> *You try going to the pharmacy with just your insurance policy document in hand and try to get medication. In the best case, they* [the pharmacy staff] *feel suspicious and so they just refuse the customer. As a rule, they always want the number of the insurance card so they can validate it electronically.*

The insurance card is needed to validate the patient's claim that they have an insurance policy. The hospital's administrative employee, Andrew, mentions this too. He says that if a patient has an AHV number, he can check it and he can also confirm whether patients are registered with a specific insurance company. The problem when a patient arrives with neither a card nor an AHV number is that:

> *We don't find these people in our searches. And then it gets difficult. Because we know he's insured but we can't verify it. And as part of our processes, well, we verify that kind of thing.*

The NGO sometimes provides a letter of guarantee to reassure the healthcare organizations' administrative employees that the costs are indeed covered. The NGO's remit may go even further to include 'advocacy', as the nurse, Melanie, explains, 'to speak for a patient, to protect him, or to elicit the best possible outcome for him or her'. At the same time, and stressing again the agency of undocumented migrants, she adds:

> *We only advocate when necessary. I mean, our people are extremely resourceful and most of them are good at getting what they need. I think it's important that we're here and that we help them. But you also need to let go. I mean, you don't want to make them dependent on you. [...] We don't want to see our patients as victims. Of course, they are to a certain extent but if you see people only as victims you lose sight of what they are actually capable of. It's kind of a fine line.*

Jonathan's story offers numerous insights into the question of how undocumented migrants are excluded from and included in communication related to their healthcare. First, it demonstrates the nature of the strategies for inclusion that are adopted by migrants when their chronic conditions worsen and they do not have the support of the NGO. Self-care strategies that threaten their health can be adopted. Inclusion is not sought via emergency care but via a risky and often futile asylum process that enables inclusion for a short period only. Still, these strategies also show a will to stay proactive when it comes to one's health. In addition, the brief inclusion in healthcare provided by the asylum application process is again contrasted with the description of care at the NGO and in its network, which offers a more lasting option.

At the turning point of Jonathan's story, we see again that administrative aspects of inclusion in healthcare, like taking out insurance, need specific arrangements. Patients are again dependent on the financial support and specialist knowledge of an NGO and a willing insurer. Jonathan's story also shows us how inclusion can remain difficult, even once a patient is insured. The problems that stem from the lack of an insurance card highlight again the importance of administration, even for such a basic need as an undocumented migrant's ability to call for an ambulance. Jonathan's story also vividly reveals that prejudice against undocumented migrants on the insurer's side, and the suspicion of administrative and medical personnel regarding uncovered costs, are tightly tangled and create difficulties that can hamper a patient's inclusion in healthcare. As in Maria's case, we can see that inclusion is dependent upon the goodwill of professionals, even if the NGO can be relied on to facilitate interactions. Still, we can see that not only the patients themselves, but also the NGO's healthcare professionals, stress the importance of giving patients the space to be agents of their own inclusion.

Jonathan's story also provides evidence to support the idea that the inclusion of undocumented migrants in healthcare must take their specific needs into account. The importance of handling the scheduling of appointments, taking care of family members, and making space to talk about problems otherwise well-hidden has been revealed in the stories of Béatrice, Peter and Maria. Jonathan's narrative takes these aspects to their extremes, showing the limits of the capacities of professionals to balance the consequences of a patient's exclusion from citizenship.

Finally, as in Maria's story, we see again that the need to be included in healthcare and the act of causing harm to one's health can come together in paradoxical ways. Ironically, getting the papers to legalize Jonathan's stay is only possible because of his exclusion from healthcare, which had physically damaged him to the point where deportation could not be carried out. Jonathan had to literally become sick enough for his status to be legalized and his healthcare financed by the state. As we already saw in Maria's story, Swiss healthcare requires a certain level of inclusion in economic or welfare systems as a prerequisite. Inclusion and exclusion start to operate paradoxically when these prerequisites are not met. In the case of undocumented migrants, these paradoxes result in lasting scars on human bodies.

6. Insurance

In this, the final chapter that deals with empirical research, we will encounter patients who identify the acquisition of insurance as their most important moment of inclusion in healthcare. We have already seen that among the total number of patients who are looked after at the NGO, and similarly among the estimated total of undocumented migrants, patients with health insurance represent a minority of around 10–20%. Anna's story will bring us back to the network of professionals that surround the NGO. It will also allow us to consider more deeply the process of obtaining insurance coverage and thus we will return to the interview with Patricia, the employee of the insurance company, and meet Brigitte, an employee of an NGO that provides care for undocumented migrants who are HIV positive. Fanny and Nicolas' stories offer insights into the value of insurance to undocumented migrants. Nicolas' case in turn will reveal more about emergency healthcare in case of accidents. His story is complemented by further contributions from Andrew, the hospital's administrative employee.

Since insurance plays such an important role in this chapter, it is worth reminding ourselves of the reasons why such a tiny fraction of undocumented migrants are insured (see also Rüefli & Hügli 2011). Besides the important financial reasons and administrative difficulties, there is another, more fundamental reason, which leaves insurers reluctant to offer their services to undocumented migrants. As we have seen, Jonathan's insurance cover was set up only at the moment there was an actual need. This is also the case for Anna, Fanny and Nicolas. Patricia says:

> Of course, an insurance company is not interested in insuring people who cause
> a lot of write-offs because [their] costs are simply not covered by their premiums.

 https://doi.org/10.11647/OBP.0139.06

This argument is not compatible with the idea that an insurance provider balances costs versus income not at an individual but at a population level. However, only obtaining insurance at the moment of need is not quite in the spirit of things either. Companies react with different strategies, as the head of the NGO, Julia, explains:

Of course, now they bring forward all sorts of reasons as to why they won't insure him, for example, they claim that 'this was the wrong form you used'. Or, in the beginning, a lot of applications just went missing.

Julia contextualises this statement by saying that it is not always 'bad will' that causes lost applications, but also the fact that sometimes the more unusual circumstances of undocumented migrants do not fit what she calls the 'insurance apparatus'. But Patricia confirms that there might be something more systematic behind the 'loss' of these applications:

And some insurers simply kick those applications into the long grass. As in, you've gone to the insurer's office three times, and you say 'I have your stamp here, you have received' — 'We have nothing'. That [application] ended in someone's rubbish bin or similar.

Sometimes, the NGO obtains legal advice to push applications through. But as David, the general practitioner who volunteers at the NGO, puts it: 'Some of them [insurers] make things so complicated, at some point you just give up'. For those insurers who cooperate, there is a delicate balance to strike between their willingness to insure and not wanting to become too attractive for NGOs taking out insurance. As the insurance employee, Patricia, explains, she sometimes initiates a conversation:

Well if there is a bit of a connection we sometimes just address them [NGOs] directly and ask if maybe one or the other case… if they're in very bad health, well, we just have a frank conversation. We state that in general we are not interested. 'We are obliged to insure them, you know that. But you have to also see our side […] wouldn't it be possible to insure this client somewhere else [with a different insurer]?' […] Of course they're not happy about this either, but there are some who, as a result, switch insurers on an annual basis. […] For us, of course, this would be ideal, if we could all take turns a bit, that way all insurers are a bit involved.

Brigitte, an employee of an AIDS Advisory Charity bureau, who also obtains insurance coverage for HIV-positive undocumented migrants, confirms this practice. She was contacted by an insurance employee who 'asked me whether we insure all of "them" with their insurance'. When asked directly whether the practice of complicating the registration process so that the patient or NGO desists, or negotiating a change of insurers, could be described as a kind of risk-selection, Patricia answers:

> *What you say is correct, there is a strong selection process. […] That's the competition of course, everyone wants to grow, everyone wants to keep their losses as low as possible.*

When it comes to asylum seekers, cantons distribute them amongst different insurers depending on the insurer's size. However, as Patricia says:

> *with the undocumented migrants, you can't do anything but talk. Because you can't control* [the insurer with whom they register].

Anna: 'Sometimes, I have a friend'

Anna is a woman in her forties. She entered Switzerland in 2011 and contacted a relative who told her that there was no way to get any healthcare without papers in Switzerland. However, when she began to earn her livelihood as a sex worker, she was informed about the NGO by a social worker. When she went to register, the general practitioner ascertained that there was a large lump in her breast. Anna, who is a mother of six, said that she had had this lump since breastfeeding her fourth child.

However, soon after, the lump started to hurt and the breast oozed liquid. Anna returned to the NGO. Echoing Béatrice, she describes having been given a hospital appointment immediately. The exams showed that she had breast cancer. She explains here that what would become her most important opportunity for inclusion was immediately put in jeopardy:

> *He said you have breast cancer. So then I started to cry because […] you know in* [my home country] *almost everyone who has this illness, their only end is death. So, from then on they started to treat me. And then I made the mistake. Because they* [the social worker's NGO] *had been paying for my health insurance, I was told I should file for asylum.*

Anna did not file an asylum request, because her relative told her there would be no chance. She regrets this today, as the NGO subsequently stopped paying her insurance and she still has to 'live in the shadows', as she puts it. The realization of how important the insurance was and is for her health and healthcare thus came to Anna retrospectively. From this moment on, she decided to pay for her insurance herself as an aging sex worker.

Still, and importantly, the insurance made it possible for her to receive cancer treatment. She had surgery and chemotherapy during 2012–2013. Anna describes the treatment as good most of the time, with medical staff acting in a caring and professional way towards her. She has a general practitioner who has been attending her since 2014, but she tries as best she can to take care of her own health. Asked what good healthcare means to her, she says:

> It's my health. So I have to take care of it. Yes, it's my health. It's my life after all.

When she feels bad, she tries to use preventative measures at home before attending a healthcare facility. She goes for walks as her general practitioner recommends, having recently been diagnosed with diabetes. As David says, a general practitioner can be an important professional for an undocumented migrant. The NGO helps its patients to contact them:

> Well we have some general practitioners where we can place them so to speak. Yes, it is rather important that they [the general practitioners] have some experience with undocumented migrants and are a bit aware as to what kind of problems that entails.

Interestingly enough he again mentions professionals who are a part of the NGO's network.

Generally, as soon as patients are insured 'we are no longer responsible [for them]', David explains. Still, as we have already seen with Peter and Jonathan, David says that patients tend to return

> because they have found they trust us, they still return [to us] with one problem or another, or to ask us to explain something.

That is also the case for Anna. She says, echoing statements made by Peter:

> I didn't hide anything from [Julia]. When I have a little problem I come and I explain to her. Sometimes, she even tells me when someone has dropped by with some clothes, [...] and I come and sort them and [...] I send them to the children.

For Anna, it is also important that she is accompanied by either the social worker or the head of the NGO whenever she has chemotherapy, or when being looked after by doctors who do not speak the Swiss national language that she speaks. All these elements contribute to her inclusion in healthcare.

On the other hand, Anna recalls an episode in which, after a session of chemotherapy, she returned to hospital because she had started to feel very ill. A mistake had been made with her medication. She says:

> *I don't even know anymore how I got out of the house to* […] *take the tram and go to the hospital, but still, I arrived there.* […] *All these parts* [points at her arms] *were already numb; I couldn't feel my feet anymore. They kept me there for eight days.*

What is striking, in parallel with Jonathan's and Béatrice's accounts, is that Anna does not mention the option of calling an ambulance either.

Still, Anna's main problem is paying the insurance premiums. The NGO has found a way to reduce the premiums for its patients (see Chapter Two for more detail about premium reductions). Nevertheless, administrative difficulties prevent them from having access to the cheapest insurance packages. Anna's serious illness likely makes it very difficult for her to continue working, which she has to do to earn enough to pay her insurance premiums. Asked about how she manages, she says: 'Sometimes, when I have a friend, I explain to him. Yes, he gives me something'. As Julia explains,

> *The high premiums that they have to pay for with their* [low] *or even non-existent wages, well,* […] *especially women enter into highly dependent relationships.* […] *Even so, a good third to a half of our people are in some way or another involved in sex work. With the corresponding illnesses.*

This statement, taken together with Anna's account about how she manages to pay her premiums, provides more evidence that undocumented migrants are sometimes forced to engage in practices that may compromise their health, in order to be included in healthcare.

When a patient requires such expensive treatment, it is very important to have insurance that covers costs from the very beginning. Inclusion has to occur at the right time. Even if it might seem obvious that insurance should cover the necessary costs right from the start, it does not always work this way in the case of undocumented migrants.

Usually, as the administrative employee of the hospital explains, people who arrive in Switzerland are obliged to organise insurance during the first three months of their stay. If they receive care during this time, while their insurance is not yet in place, costs are covered retrospectively as soon as the contract is signed. The insurance in turn will fix the start of the contract at the moment the person has registered at a municipality.

But in the case of undocumented migrants, it is not possible to know whether the individual really intends to stay. As a result, the insurance provider has to bear the risk of signing contracts with clients who might have only entered the country in order to get treatment. In such a case the insurance company can refuse to sign the contract, or rescind the contract when the individual leaves the country. Because of this, Patricia states, the company is 'very sensitive to the fact, if there's a recent hospital admission' just after a contract has been taken out. On the other hand, it also might be that the insured undocumented migrant has already been in the country for years. In this case, as Patricia explains:

> there's an article [in law] *that states — this applies specifically to people who are in Switzerland, who are in a bit of a, let's call it a grey area — that, in those cases, we can rely on* [the fact] *that the date that counts is the date on which we receive the insurance document.* [...] *So, nothing is done retroactively.*

Indeed, the *Verordnung über die Krankenversicherung* (KVV) states that if a person registers later than three months after their arrival, the insurance starts only at the moment of the registration (Art. 7 al. 1). Also, the insurer can demand a supplementary premium (Art. 8). Julia relates a case in which an insurance company made a patient pay a month's premium as a supplement, but without covering expenses that had arisen during this time. As she put it: 'You pay an empty premium'. In this case, the NGO ended up paying the uncovered care costs of CHF 400; 4/5 of the annual budget for one patient.

Brigitte, the employee of the NGO caring for HIV-positive undocumented migrants, says that this practice is rather recent. In order not to generate costs that would not be covered by insurance, she asks doctors not to start HIV treatment as soon as the diagnosis is made, even if there is some urgency, especially when the HIV is already in a progressive state. Rather, doctors should wait until the insurance is certain to be valid:

We informed [the doctors] *that their medical standards and the actual possibilities do not always coincide.*

The most salient aspects of Anna's story are the difficulties that her inclusion in healthcare cause her. Once more, an undocumented migrant is included in healthcare at the cost of harm to her health, as well as being heavily dependent upon other people. And while such difficulties might also affect Swiss citizens, being undocumented exacerbates these problems, due to the absence of any legal, social and working security entitlements. Taking financial responsibility for her inclusion in healthcare is, first and foremost, a huge burden for Anna. Her situation is such that even if she still tries to actively care for her health, her opportunities to do so have become very restricted. The spectres of despair and hopelessness pervade the whole interview.

The debate about the exact point at which insurance coverage begins shows once again the extent to which undocumented migrants are dependent on the NGO to ensure that all the administrative procedures are carried out correctly. These are also closely tied to financial aspects of inclusion in healthcare-related communications and the healthcare system itself, governed by interactions with medical personnel. This close entanglement between the financial, administrative and care aspects of inclusion might result in important treatments being postponed.

While Anna's treatment for her breast cancer is certainly very important to her health, there are still problematic gaps in her inclusion when it comes to her ability to access help in emergency situations. Anna also depends on the help of NGOs. Just like Peter, Maria and Jonathan, Anna stresses the importance of the NGO in maintaining her healthcare in a wider sense, despite having a family doctor who sees her.

Fanny: 'I can just make an appointment'

Fanny, a woman in her late twenties, has now been living in Switzerland for about twelve years. At the time of her arrival, like Jonathan and Maria, though in better health and still a minor, she enrolled in an asylum process. During this time, she learned one of the national languages, which she now speaks fluently. At that time, she also had a family doctor at her side who regularly examined her one remaining kidney. As she explains, she lost the other one in her home country, while undergoing surgery because of a kidney stone:

> *And then they said, now there's nothing we can do. This kidney [...], the right one, so this side, they removed everything.*

Fanny's asylum request was turned down in 2007, but she decided to stay in Switzerland. She was in the company of compatriots during her migration and from the very beginning of her stay. Via this diaspora community, she found a cleaning job that enabled her to afford housing and food. When it came to her health, Fanny medicated herself with some paracetamol when she experienced pain. She expresses concerns about this kind of self-medication:

> *I also have stomach pain, many [times], and I have always taken medicine, but that's not good either, no? I don't know if I can just take this medicine, or, I don't know. And then I still have such strong pain.*

Then, in 2012, she fell pregnant. Having had no examinations during her pregnancy, she decided, towards the ninth month of her term, to undergo the asylum process for a second time, as she explains:

> *Because, it's difficult. When you are illegal in Switzerland to have a baby you have to pay [so] much, and you have to work [so] much [...]. That's why I made a second request.*

Fanny explains that she only felt safe to begin the asylum process again because she was so heavily pregnant that she was sure she would not be deported. At the end of this second asylum attempt, she went into hiding once more, this time with her newborn child.

It was during her second pregnancy in 2015 that Fanny was finally introduced to the NGO by a friend. All pregnant patients attending the NGO are urged to take out insurance, and Julia stresses that she does not want a 'parallel universe' of healthcare for undocumented migrants and deplores any situation in which a patient remains without insurance. Fanny did not even know she was entitled to take out insurance, but once this was established she was very pleased to have it. She is in a less financially precarious situation than Anna, and so she focuses most of all on its organizational and administrative advantages. She can go 'to the women's clinic, just normal'. She continues:

Now that I pay the insurance every month and when I have pain somewhere, then I go, then [there] *is no problem.* […] *Then I have no worries, right. When I have pain or something, I don't have to think, ah, what should I do or something. I can just make an appointment.* [It] *is easier and much better.*

Fanny stresses the value of the insurance again in the following statement, comparing her current situation to that in her home country:

When I go to hospital or the like [in my home country], *I always heard them talking, they wanted money. We have to give something, right. And then they do it. But if we don't give anything or so, then they didn't want to. No, that is different, right, here in Switzerland they don't do this, right. When I go to hospital, I give money to nobody.*

We see similarities here to Béatrice's experience, when she talked about the relief of not having to incentivise every medical interaction with some sort of payment. Paying for and receiving care are social relations enacted at different points in time and with different organizations. The insurance means that Fanny's inclusion in healthcare is independent from any individual's goodwill or corruptibility. It allows her to take part in a process in which personal negotiation and bargaining are not necessary.

Asked about how she finances the insurance, Fanny just says that she has to 'work a lot' in order to pay the premiums. Her two children are not insured, but get some basic care at the NGO. Even Fanny, who is at this point able to handle most of her interactions with healthcare organizations herself, states that the NGO gives the hospital a call before she visits, 'so then they don't ask too many questions'.

With Fanny's story we have encountered a case that, although more turbulent than Anna's in some respects, shows clearly how migrants can create a significant amount of space for autonomous inclusion and how much they value this autonomy. For Fanny, it seems, the insurance gives her a sense of having a certain right to exist and to be recognized in Switzerland, if not as citizen, then at least as a patient. Again, contact with the diaspora and inclusion in a labour market, however precarious, allow Fanny to obtain healthcare relatively independently.

On the other hand, Fanny's case shows once more what kind of inclusion undocumented migrants can obtain while remaining excluded from charitable organizations and insurance. To file an asylum request is a marginalizing and risky strategy for inclusion in healthcare.

Nicolas: 'I know I have to pay because I know why'

Nicolas came to Switzerland in 2003 after abandoning his studies in Germany for financial reasons. He always thought that maybe he could earn enough money to finish his studies, but he was never able to save anything on the side. Still, of all the patients discussed in this book, he is financially probably the most secure. He works in agriculture and on building sites, as he explains:

> *I know maybe a good ten or fifteen people; sometimes I work with people like that. Sometimes he says no, this time there's no work, but I'll call you. So sometimes they call.*

Nicolas' first experience with health issues in Switzerland is directly related to one of his jobs. Working on a building site, while not yet having taken out insurance, he has an accident and hurts his knee:

> *There was a lady [...] she says 'mister mister hello what's up', and I say 'listen, I fell, I don't know what's up'. She said 'my husband is ambulance driver' [...] and she called and he came with the ambulance and he put a thing like this, like ice.*

Despite receiving this first aid, Nicolas does not let the driver take him to hospital. He instead says he wants to go home, as it is already late. He also repeats twice that he 'doesn't know anybody' in the hospital. The fear of going to an emergency unit because he does not know anybody echoes the dependency on personal connections that has already been stated by other patients. Again, it seems that undocumented migrants have to rely so heavily on personal and informal relationships that they do not dare to interact with organizations where no such connections exist. Only the next day, when the knee has swollen even more, is Nicolas willing to go to the hospital. His boss picks him up in a car, drives him to the unit and pays for the care given.

For Nicolas, things are uneventful after this incident until his sight starts to trouble him. Still not insured, he is examined by an ophthalmologist. When describing this incident, Nicolas says 'I paid him for nothing'. The doctor tells him that there's nothing wrong and that he just should get new glasses. Nicolas continues:

> *I said 'listen, I tell you the truth. I trust you. I don't have papers here in Switzerland. How much does this cost?' He said '500 francs'. I said [...] 'can*

*you, can you wait a little moment, for example, some days, a week?' He said
'listen, you have to pay now'. [...] Maybe he is stressed, maybe he thinks I won't
pay.*

Nicolas therefore has to pay CHF 500 for a diagnosis he suspects to be
wrong and, as the doctor wants the money at once, he bargains with an
employer in order to get an advance on his salary.

Nicolas then turns to another professional, who tells him that he does
indeed need surgery on his eyes and should take out insurance. We will
come back to the details about how Nicolas obtains and affords this
insurance. For now, suffice it to say that with the contract taken out in
2010, he can get the surgery he needs. He says he was afraid during the
first surgery, which is reminiscent of Peter's experience. Both men know
that surgeries in their countries of origin can be very risky procedures,
potentially accompanied by dangerous complications. Nicolas describes
how the hospital personnel calmed him and informed him about every
step taken. He is very happy with the results and with the operation on
the second eye, as he says, 'I go there easy and hop hop, no problem'.
Like Fanny, he values the insurance a great deal:

*The insurance, that works very well here, that helps a lot. [...] And I know I have
to pay because I know why.*

He does his best to pay the premiums on time. When things get tight
with money, he can sometimes get an advance from one of his employers
and 'sometimes I don't eat'. We encounter here another example of
inclusion in healthcare creating a need for behaviour that threatens the
patient's health. On one occasion, Nicolas ends up calling the insurance
company:

*Once I called them, they sent me a letter: if you don't pay — police. I said,
'Listen, I'm not like you. You have a salary, I don't. I work a bit here and there
and then I don't work for two or three months, it depends'. Ah, he understood.
'Listen, when I have [a] delay [...] I pay it anyway'.*

Nicolas again stresses the importance of insurance in his next statement,
though adding at the same time a bleaker comment:

*The insurance is obligatory because sometimes I do dangerous work. So it has
to be done. [...] The problem, when I have no work, how do I pay? I have to take
any kind of work I can get.*

Nicolas's statements reinforce the pattern seen in Anna's story, in which friends helped to pay for her insurance and she therefore developed dependent relationships common amongst undocumented migrants in order to pay premiums. Again, we see how healthcare has to tackle problems that, to a great extent, have been caused by the financial difficulties encountered during the process of gaining inclusion in healthcare. To 'know why you have to pay' in Nicolas's case therefore means knowing you have to pay because you know you are at the risk of injuries. These injuries are caused by the hard and risky physical work you have to carry out in order to be able to pay for the insurance in the first place.

To acquire and maintain health insurance also involves a lot of administrative work for Nicolas. As soon as the doctor tells him that he needs insurance, he turns to a social worker he happens to know. The social worker does some research and finally tells him that he needs a 'legal' person whom he trusts and who trusts him, so that financial transactions and correspondence can take place. After he finds this person, whom Nicolas describes as a good friend, the three of them meet up and organize an appointment at an insurance company:

> *Because she* [his friend] *made the bank account and all, and then every time I call or I send an SMS like this, I say, 'Listen, are there any bills?'* [...] *She says yes. Ok, I'll come at once. And then, sometimes, I don't find her at home, so I put the money in an envelope for her. And then she organizes everything.*

To 'organize everything' means, for example, to try to get a premium reduction and to try to ensure the provision of the canton's contribution in case of hospital stays. As Patricia explains, hospitals who cannot assign patients to a certain canton, because they are not registered, tend to send the whole bill to the insurance company, while usually the canton has to pay 55% of a hospital stay. Patricia adds: 'Usually, it's the institution [e.g. an NGO] that checks whom one can turn to'.

As we saw in the introduction to this study, Nicolas did not receive an insurance card:

> *I don't have an insurance card, but with the* [insurance] *number they find it. Now, this works at* [one particular hospital], *but the other hospitals I don't know.*

The interesting part of this statement is that Nicolas mentions a specific hospital, at which he had his eye surgery. Other hospitals, such as the one I accompanied him to, do not have him registered as a patient and therefore, being unable to verify his insurance without a card, are reluctant to register him.

Finally, the biggest remaining problem for Nicolas is his lack of papers. This is a particular difficulty. Given his country of origin, he has very little chance of legalizing his status in Switzerland. At the same time, he cannot return. Because there is no repatriation agreement between Switzerland and the country in question, the government there simply refuses to take back any undocumented migrants. As Julia puts it:

> *It's like they belong nowhere. Switzerland doesn't want them and* [Nicolas' country of origin] *doesn't want them anymore either.*

For undocumented migrants in this situation, encounters with the police end up being pointless, but can still have serious repercussions, as Julia explains:

> *Sometimes they end up in administrative detention because they were stopped by police. And because they can't be deported, they can just keep them there for a few months and then they put them back on the street.*

Being in prison for months can easily result in loss of work, housing and contacts. Having lived under these threats for fifteen years now, Nicolas, like Maria, says that he does not tell people about his problems. He states that he is otherwise in good health, he does a lot of exercise to stay healthy and to avoid thinking too much about his problems. He can always rely on the NGO when he needs to talk. But he adds:

> *I don't sleep when I think, I don't sleep how I should, really. Even when I spend the whole day outside, I do sport, but there's always a nightmare because of* [lacking papers]. *Believe me, sometimes I cry.*

Nicolas's story also returns us to the issues surrounding emergency care, this time in the context of a work accident. Regardless of the issue of cost, the fear of being exposed due to a lack of personal connections often holds undocumented migrants back from attending emergency care, as we have already seen. In the case of a work accident in a black market setting, for instance, this fear is not completely unfounded. As Andrew, the hospital's administrative employee, confirms:

> *Well it does happen that they are 'visiting' someone on the construction site. And then they have an accident. And then we see what we can do with the police.*

Julia relates this as a situation of conflicting loyalties:

> *In some way, they* [the hospital's employees] *have a conflicting task. On the one hand, to protect the client, and on the other hand, to collaborate with the authorities.*

From Andrew's perspective, these different loyalties can clash in a paradoxical way. Sometimes, Andrew, himself a Swiss citizen, thinks it might be better for the patient to force their employer to live up to their legal responsibilities and provide healthcare, even if this results in the patient losing their permit to stay in the country.[1] As Andrew puts it:

> *There's the question as to what's more important. In this particular situation, it's probably a matter of weighing things up. And depending on the severity of* [the accident] *it's certainly better for the patient to accept the consequences.*

Nicolas' case effectively demonstrates how undocumented migrants try to deal with incidents of ill health when they are broadly excluded from healthcare. There are options, such as simply to ignore a problem, or to depend on an employer to provide transport to and payment for treatment, but this carries the risk of arousing the suspicion of healthcare professionals about one's legal status and/or financial precarity. We see again that the fear of being exposed and/or being burdened with very high costs of care excludes migrants like Nicolas from emergency departments.

Nicolas's story also demonstrates, once more, the benefits that insurance can bring for undocumented migrants, in contrast to the difficulty of their attempts to be included in healthcare without it. It must be understood, however, that this value also carries a high

---

1   As soon as a patient who has had an accident declares himself to be employed — whether legally or on the black market — his employer's insurance has to bear the cost of his healthcare. But by declaring themselves to be illegally employed, undocumented migrants expose themselves and are deported after treatment.

price — a substantial financial burden, but also the cost to one's health that is often inflicted by attempts to afford insurance.

We also see the lengths to which undocumented migrants can go to continue their participation in an insurance scheme, and how, despite this effort, they usually remain dependent upon someone else, who functions as an addressee and bank account holder. Being able to receive treatment from medical personnel is not assured even then, because exclusion at the hospital is a potential issue if the patient is not backed by an organization like the NGO.

7. Healthcare for undocumented migrants

Dynamics of inclusion and exclusion

The preceding chapters have outlined three core moments of inclusion in healthcare that can be experienced by undocumented migrants, along with their preconditions and consequences. This section reviews those moments, preconditions and consequences, and then contrasts them with situations in which patients remain excluded from communication related to or directly concerning healthcare.

Firstly, as we have seen with Suzanne's story, settling in is an important moment of inclusion. However, it is contingent upon preconditions, which typically include knowing somebody in the country of arrival and having migrated in order to seek a different life or work, rather than out of sheer personal distress or danger caused by sickness, war or torture, as was the case for Jonathan or Maria.

Having contacts within a diaspora community who can assist a new arrival to find housing and work is a great advantage, enabling an undocumented migrant to build a life that they find relatively satisfying and healthy, even if certain issues continue to weigh on them. Opportunities to be proactive about one's own situation allow one to address minor health issues and soothe some of the difficulties of an undocumented life. As we have seen, these difficulties are first and foremost due to undocumented status itself, which makes both work and family life insecure and brings with it a fear of discovery (see also

 https://doi.org/10.11647/OBP.0139.07

Wysmüller & Efionayi-Mäder 2011:44; Biswas et al. 2011; Achermann et al. 2006). The importance of good health in maintaining a decent quality of life in such a stressful situation, and the fragility of this kind of inclusion, are in turn demonstrated by cases in which serious health issues arose and difficult social situations had an impact on a person's health and healthcare.

The second important moment of inclusion is the point of initial contact with the NGO and its network. However, some social connections with a diaspora community, with social workers or with other NGOs are necessary to discover it, as we have seen with Jonathan and Fanny for example. Informal knowledge is thus essential, as also described by Huschke (2014) in reference to Berlin and Devillanova (2008) in relation to Milan.

Enabling inclusion in healthcare in specific ways is a core competency of the NGO, making it an important actor in this respect. Administrative processes are tailored as much as possible to fit the specific situations of undocumented migrants, as illustrated by Béatrice's account. Furthermore, the NGO helps migrants to bear the burden of particular difficulties with inclusion that result from ideological, administrative and financial dependence on medical and insurance professionals, with the result that the NGO is, to a certain extent, involved in these difficulties itself. If needed, the NGO not only provides a space in which patients can receive healthcare, but also offers them opportunities to address the health issues of their families back home and to discuss the difficulties of an undocumented life, as Peter's account has shown.

One consequence of being included in healthcare at the NGO and its network is that migrants can receive at least some care at a reduced cost, or acquire treatment for conditions that had remained undiagnosed in the mainstream system. However, the undocumented migrants also become dependent on a charitable organization. Inclusion is therefore organized in the separate framework of a parallel healthcare system, one that necessarily lags behind the mainstream structure that is accessible to legal residents. When undocumented migrants who have not discovered the NGO experience health issues, they sometimes try to ignore the problem for as long as possible, as Maria's story demonstrated (see also Biswas et al. 2011 and Wolff et al. 2008). Finally, in order to receive some sort of assistance with their health, they may seek to be included in the healthcare system in ways that are marginalizing and risky, such as telling lies in order to receive medication. They sometimes turn to futile and even perilous asylum procedures, like Jonathan and Fanny, and are likely to engage in practices that actually harm their health (for other examples of such strategies see also Achermann et al. 2006:147ff; Huschke 2014; Roura et al. 2015). Inclusion in the emergency services is typically only sought after a trusted person has reassured the patient that they can use these services safely. In contrast to the professionals' view (confirmed by Dauvin et al. 2012) that even without insurance, inclusion at emergency units is possible, undocumented migrants are often excluded in practice by their fear of incurring costs they will not be able to pay, and chiefly by the dread of their status being exposed, as Nicolas' account has shown. Legal entitlement does not equate to actual inclusion into healthcare. In some countries (Poduval et al. 2015; and to a certain extent Biswas et al. 2011), patients seem to have a better understanding of the healthcare services they are entitled to access. This finding strengthens the idea that inclusion is as contingent on the circumstances and actions of the patient as on the actions of the professionals concerned. Inclusion is indeed a social relation and not an individual feature or a property of organizations.

A third key moment of inclusion in healthcare is acquiring insurance. This allows access to more expensive and longer-term treatments. More than that, insurance can give the undocumented migrant a sense of having an active role in achieving their inclusion in healthcare, and the ability to interact (in certain cases quite autonomously) with the different actors related to their care. As Laranché explains in her study, and has we have seen in Fanny's story, the knowledge that one has a right to healthcare, and being entitled to this right by contract, can be a 'means of becoming recognized as existing' (Laranché 2012:862).

But again, support from an NGO or a person who possesses specialised knowledge, such as a social worker, is essential to be able to take out insurance. To hold insurance, one again needs to be settled, to have the help of trusted people and above all to have some money on hand.

Acquiring insurance, as a single moment and as a lasting relationship of inclusion, can result in patients being forced into a position of financial dependence on family, friends, acquaintances, clients or employers, as Maria's and Nicolas' stories demonstrated. The financial demands and related stresses involved with maintaining insurance payments can in themselves pose a substantial threat to good health. As Fleischmann puts it, financial pressures 'perpetuate the cycle of harsh work conditions and deteriorating health' (2012:93). To be involved in the official labour market, or to have access to the welfare state via citizenship, prove to be — frequently unspoken — prerequisites to obtaining healthcare. And yet, having taken out insurance, patients are still at risk of being excluded from healthcare facilities, unless they have people to accompany them or organizations to advocate for them. Underuse of medical services is therefore not only, as Hügli & Rüfli (2011:39) state, due to patients not daring to use services, but also due to some services excluding patients. As Dauvin et al. (2012) have asserted in the context of the British healthcare system, this makes it difficult for professionals to refer patients to other healthcare facilities, if the patients plan to attend those facilities on their own. Biswas et al. (2011) confirm the importance of knowing citizens in order to obtain healthcare in Denmark.

However, a lack of insurance can also be a serious impediment to health, tying patients to the limited possibilities of paying for care themselves or forcing them to rely on the restricted financial resources of a charitable organization.

All these moments of inclusion in healthcare function to improve the life and health of patients, in contrast to those situations in which patients are only able to achieve partial inclusion or are even excluded completely from healthcare. Such situations exacerbate bad health or cause patients to seek out marginalizing and risky ways of obtaining healthcare.

Furthermore, in all these moments of inclusion, certain preconditions have to be fulfilled, such as knowing someone in the country of arrival, being able to work and having the opportunities to work. It is necessary to have local connections to get to the NGO and to take out insurance. Regarding insurance, having enough paid work is an indispensable prerequisite. Inclusion in healthcare thus requires inclusion in the social systems of diaspora communities and inclusion in an economic system.

Finally, whatever steps patients and professionals undertake, there are significant limitations on the inclusion of undocumented migrants in healthcare. If patients are uninsured, diagnosis and treatment are limited to the strictly necessary, unless professionals are willing to give more time out of the goodness of their hearts. Important health problems sometimes simply cannot be addressed, as we have seen in Maria's case. When patients have insurance, inclusion is still not available at the same level as for Swiss citizens, as advocacy is still needed. Furthermore, to achieve inclusion, patients are frequently forced to accept occupational health risks at disproportionate levels compared to Swiss citizens. Exclusion from the nation state and systems of citizenship therefore causes exclusion or precarity of inclusion in healthcare: exclusions foster further exclusions. Thus, our research confirms the idea that being undocumented is a social determinant of health on its own (Martinez et al. 2015; Castaneda 2009, Affronti et al. 2013; Kuehne et al. 2015, Fleischmann 2012). In a systems theory approach this 'spillover' between systems — the determination of healthcare and health by legal status — is seen as a contradiction, given that the systems see themselves as autonomous and independent from each other. For instance, in Switzerland, access to healthcare is (as we have seen in Chapter Two) decoupled from citizenship in the system's own formal description. In practice however, in the operative enactment of communication, this is not the case. Stichweh refers to such effects as 'corrupt local structural coupling'[1] between systems (2005:175f). As a consequence, patients are often pushed into a parallel healthcare system, such as that offered by the NGO and its network. Integrative inclusion seems to be much less common than separating inclusion, to lean once again on Stichweh's (2007) terminology.

Contexts and dimensions of inclusion and exclusion

As may be increasingly apparent to the reader, all these moments can lead to inclusion or exclusion in various social contexts. Three main contexts have appeared in the material gathered:

1. the economic context, concerning financial aspects,
2. the organizational/administrative context,
3. the treatment context.

---

1   'korrupte lokale strukturelle Kopplungen'.

Financial aspects are tied to inclusion in the economy as a functional system: work brings with it the ability to mediate social relations through monetary payment. Organizational and administrative contexts refer to an individual's inclusion in organizations, be they insurance or healthcare organizations. Lastly, contexts of treatment concern inclusion in the system of healthcare as a functional social system.

When discussing these three contexts, three important dimensions of inclusion and exclusion become evident. These dimensions point towards a shared culture and shared values between both undocumented migrants and the professionals caring for them. The three dimensions concern:

1. the question of whether inclusion can only be achieved in the short term, or whether it can be stabilized for a longer period;

2. the question of how much dependence inclusion brings with it, or of how much independence and self-determination it allows;

3. the question of whether inclusion leads to the recognition and addressing of the specific conditions in which undocumented migrants live, or not.

Each context mentioned above can be related to these dimensions of inclusion and exclusion. For example, financial inclusion can be said to be achieved over a longer or shorter period; it can make dependence greater or smaller; it can take into account or ignore the situation of undocumented migrants. The same holds true for the other two contexts.

While going through these contexts and dimensions, it will once again become evident how tightly they are interlinked and how they are also tied to legal status and thus to policies concerning undocumented migration and healthcare. It would be interesting to compare these findings with stories of other vulnerable populations and see where similarities and differences appear. It is striking that, while the interviewed patients had very diverse migration backgrounds and origins that were widely spread across the globe, it is still possible to identify common dimensions concerning inclusion and exclusion. Much more than any regional culture, it seems to be the fact of being undocumented itself that creates a specific environment and culture and brings forward specific needs (for a similar insight in quantitative studies concerning migrants in general see Arevalo et al. 2015 and Ikram et al. 2015).

Firstly, financial inclusion is affected by the fact that undocumented migrants are frequently employed on the black market, leading to very low and irregular incomes. The consequent lack of any employment protection leaves them with little leverage when it comes to negotiating for salaries, notice periods, or protection in case of accident, sickness or maternity. While financial instability is certainly also an issue among poorer Swiss citizens, being undocumented exacerbates these problems, as has been proposed by Fleischmann et al. (2015). All care, be it paid out of pocket or covered by insurance, is constantly threatened by the potential interruption of payment due to loss of work, sickness or inadequate wages.

Paying for care out of pocket or paying for insurance both result in dependence. As previously stated, undocumented migrants are likely to be pushed into jobs that are dangerous to their health due to financial pressures arising from the high cost of healthcare. They are either vulnerable to exploitation by unscrupulous employers or acquaintances, or forced to rely on charity. Furthermore, in social systems theory, money is conceived as a medium of communication in the economic system (Luhmann 1997). As such, money facilitates communication, which in the economic system consists mostly of financial exchanges. It seems that in the absence of such a medium, emotions, pity and personal concern are used as a substitute. Patients, as well as NGOs, end up begging for treatment at reduced prices. The system gives no consideration to the circumstances of migrants' lives, as they strive to achieve financial inclusion in healthcare.

Switzerland is one of the European countries with the highest out-of-pocket contribution rate when it comes to healthcare (De Pietro et al. 2015:229ff). In the cases examined in this study, the effect that being undocumented has on a person's healthcare — this 'corrupt local coupling' — is strongly linked to the financial context. However, Swiss policies regarding healthcare for undocumented migrants widely ignore this fact; despite reduced insurance premiums, patients often face insurmountably high costs, and an approach that takes this into account is currently only being realized in Lausanne and Geneva. In an interesting article, Britz and McKee (2015) investigate the consequences of charging migrants for healthcare in the UK. Experts feared that such a practice would exacerbate existing barriers and generate increased costs. The present study has revealed real-life examples of what it means for undocumented migrants to be charged financially for healthcare; even in the absence of a full economic evaluation, the results, to put it mildly, do not suggest that imitation of this model is to be encouraged.

Secondly, administrative inclusion is affected by the difficulty of providing proof of residency, lack of registration, the need for compliance with special data protection rules, and practical issues such as the requirement to attend appointments at the allocated time, which is often unworkable for people leading a precarious existence. Even in emergency situations, inclusion in healthcare is threatened by administrative exclusion, such as insurance companies failing to issue cards to undocumented migrants. As Laranché (2012) shows in France, Fleischmann (2015:92) in Israel, and as the present study has shown in Switzerland, such administrative exclusion is mentioned repeatedly in the statements of undocumented migrants, who think they are not entitled to emergency care.

These administrative aspects of inclusion are also affected by financial aspects. As we have seen, insurance companies practice exclusion via risk selection, or else find legal loopholes to avoid covering costs and thereby financially exclude patients before their treatment can begin. We have encountered hospitals that are driven to be financially profitable and have therefore chosen to operate along managerial lines and require their staff to react with suspicion and block procedures if in doubt about coverage of costs. An interesting question for further research could be to ask, again following Laranché's (2012) approach, how discourses and politico-legal structures that relate to undocumented migrants in Switzerland shape such organizational arrangements and practices of inclusion and exclusion.

As we have seen, it is possible to set up administrative inclusion in a way that makes it responsive to the situations and specific needs of undocumented migrants. However, as things stand, patients are reliant on special knowledge that they are unable to access without outside help. NGOs, having such knowledge at their disposal, navigate grey areas where official procedures are replaced by personal connections, goodwill and special arrangements.

Administrative exclusion is thus a concern for both uninsured and insured undocumented migrants. The exclusion of the latter is especially questionable in terms of the ethics of equality. Indeed, undocumented migrants who become insured have to put in a much greater effort than legal residents, as illustrated by numerous examples in this study. They are also the ones who continue to need informal help in order to claim the rights they pay for so dearly.

Thirdly, when we consider healthcare as the interaction between medical professionals and patients, we have seen that continuity is possible if trust can be built up and administrative and financial inclusion achieved. Sometimes, especially if the health issue is physical and can be cured quite straightforwardly with the appropriate treatment, inclusion need not be tailored to the particular situation of undocumented migrants — in other words, it can be the same as the care provided to all other patients. One possible exception is that additional explanations about treatments might be needed, taking into account differing conditions in migrants' countries of origin. It is clear that health issues that are more closely linked to the legal status of undocumented migrants need to be addressed in a specific way that goes beyond what healthcare in a narrower sense might encompass, as is already the case in some instances, notably at the NGO (see Baldassar et al. 2016 for care in transnational families). For professionals who lack sensitivity to such issues, the provision of healthcare to undocumented migrants might, at times, become a difficult task. Confirming this finding, Duvin et al. (2012) state that 'communication barriers' were reported to be a more significant obstacle to obtaining primary healthcare than for emergency services.

It must be said again that, even with all the efforts made by patients and healthcare professionals, the fundamental problem, the lack of documentation, cannot be resolved in most cases. If it is resolved, this is accomplished only after long years of unnecessary difficulties and suffering.

These tightly interlocking factors that influence inclusion support the argument that inclusion is a multidimensional process. It means much more than simply being given the chance to interact with medical staff. In this regard, research should focus not only on medical personnel, but also on those who hold administrative and managerial roles. As we have seen, these gatekeepers prove to be, in some circumstances at least, as important for inclusion in healthcare as nurses and doctors. Administrative staff might need to have even more sensitivity to specific conditions and circumstances than medical staff.

Comparisons with other patient groups may show important differences in the mechanisms of inclusion. That said, it could be interesting not only to advocate a 'patient centred' approach to the access and use of healthcare (Levesque et al. 2013), but to take the idea even further, with a 'patient informed' approach to inclusion into the social systems related to healthcare.

Legal status, healthcare and health

Summing up the moments, preconditions, and consequences of healthcare inclusion and exclusion, we can see that:

Addressing financial aspects of inclusion, be it by paying out of pocket, by bargaining with a restricted and dependent NGO, or by buying insurance, is always difficult in the long term. These strategies often pose a threat to the patients' health, and only in rare cases operate as a boost to self-esteem. Patients can be included financially — but at a very high cost to their financial and social circumstances, and even their health.

Adapting administrative aspects of inclusion to the needs of undocumented migrants is possible. However, such adaptations are only rarely made by health insurers and care facilities. The situation is similarly unsatisfactory for both uninsured undocumented migrants in need of emergency care and insured undocumented migrants in need of regular healthcare. This leaves patients dependent for administrative inclusion on charitable organizations and trusted individuals.

Finally, in order to give treatment to undocumented migrants, it is not always mandatory, but sometimes desirable, to adapt the process so that it addresses at least some of the specific health issues that affect them. This task is mostly left to specialized charitable organizations and their volunteer networks.

The inclusion of undocumented migrants in healthcare in Switzerland remains partial and precarious. Exclusion is a reality and an ever-present threat, even while both patients and professionals are making every possible effort to achieve inclusion. Undocumented migrants are included in some aspects of healthcare, but only by paying a high price. Their inclusion is partial and they are excluded from some aspects of care, notwithstanding entitlements such as insurance. The health and healthcare of undocumented migrants are therefore deeply affected by their legal status. A discussion about whether this makes sense in political, economic and ethical terms is urgently needed in Switzerland — and beyond.

8. Literature

Achermann, C., et al., *Migration, Prekarität und Gesundheit. Ressourcen und Risiken von vorläufig Aufgenommenen und Sans-Papier in Genf und Zürich*, Neuchâtel: SFM Studien 41 2006.

Affronti, M., et al., "The Health of Irregular and Illegal Migrants: Analysis of Day-Hospital Admissions in a Department of Migration Medicine", *Internal and Emergency Medicine* 8 (2013), pp. 561–66, http://doi.org/10.1007/s11739-011-0635-2

Altenburg, F., "Health Services for Undocumented Migrants in Europe: An Overview", in G. Biffl, et al. (ed.), *Migration and Health in Nowhereland: Access of Undocumented Migrants to Work and Health Care in Europe*, Bad Vöslau: OMNIUM 2012, pp. 99–108, http://ec.europa.eu/chafea/documents/news/Book_NowHerecare.pdf

Anlaufstelle für Sans Papiers, *Leben und Arbeiten im Schatten. Die Erste Detaillierte Umfrage zu den Lebens- und Arbeitsbedingungen von Sans-Papiers in der Deutschschweiz*, Basel: Anlaufstelle für Sans Papiers 2004.

Arlettaz, S., "Saisonniers", in *Historisches Lexikon der Schweiz* (2012), http://www.hls-dhs-dss.ch/textes/d/D25738.php

Arevalo, S. P., et al., "Beyond Cultural Factors to Understand Immigrant Mental Health: Neighborhood Ethnic Density and the Moderating Role of Pre-migration and Post-migration Factors", *Social Science & Medicine* 138 (2015), pp. 91–100, http://doi.org/10.1016/j.socscimed.2015.05.040

Baldassar, L., et al., "Transnational Families, Care and Wellbeing", inThomas, F. (ed.), *Handbook of Migration and Health*, Cheltenham: Edward Elgar Publishing 2016, pp. 477–97.

Biffl, G., et al. (eds.), *Migration and Health in Nowhereland: Access of Undocumented Migrants to Work and Health Care in Europe*, Bad Vöslau: OMNIUM 2012.

Bilger, V., et al., *Health Care for Undocumented Migrants in Switzerland. Policies — People — Practices*, Wien: International Center for Migration Policy Development 2011, https://www.unine.ch/files/live/sites/sfm/files/nouvelles publications/Booklet-Publikation_FINAL_03082011_A5.pdf

Biswas, D., et al., "Access to Health Care for Undocumented Migrants from a Humanitarian Rights Perspective: A Comparative study of Denmark, Sweden and the Netherlands", *Health and Human Rights* 14.2 (2012), pp. 49–60.

Biswas, D. et al., "Access to Healthcare and Alternative Health-Seeking Strategies among Undocumented Migrants in Denmark", *BMC Public Health* 11.560 (2011), https://doi.org/10.1186/1471-2458-11-560

Bivins, R., *Contagious Communities. Medicine, Migration & the NHS in Post War Britain*, Oxford: Oxford University Press, 2015.

Björngren-Cuadra, C., and S. Cattacin, *Policies on Healthcare for Undocumented Migrants in the EU-27 and Switzerland: Towards a Comparative Framework. Summary Report*, 2nd edn., Malmö, 2011.

Björngren-Cuadra, C., "Policy Towards Undocumented Migrants of the EU 27", in G. Biffl, et al. (eds.), *Migration and Health in Nowhereland: Access of Undocumented Migrants to Work and Health Care in Europe*, Bad Vöslau: OMNIUM 2012, pp. 109–32.

Bloch, A., et al., *Sans Papiers: The Social and Economic Lives of Young Undocumented Migrants*, London: Pluto Press 2014.

Bodenmann, P., et al., "Screening for Latent Tuberculosis Infection Among Undocumented Immigrants in Swiss Healthcare Centres", *BMC Infectious Diseases* 9.34 (2009), http://doi.org/10.1186/1471-2334-9-34

Bommes, M. and V. Tacke, "Arbeit als Inklusionsmedium Moderner Organisationen", in V. Tacke, (ed.), *Organisation und Gesellschaftliche Differenzierung*, Wiesbaden: Westdeutscher Verlag 2001, pp. 61–83.

Britz, J. B. and M. McKee, "Charging Migrants for Health Care Could Compromise Public Health and Increase Costs for the NHS", *The Journal of Public Health* 38.2 (2015), pp. 384–90, http://doi.org/10.1093/pubmed/fdv043

Bundesamt für Sozialversicherungen: Versicherungspflicht der Sans-papiers, Weisung vom 19, Dezember 2002, Kreisschreiben 2.10, Bern: BSV 2002.

Bundesgesetz über den Allgemeinen Teil des Sozialversicherungsrechts vom 6. Oktober 2000 (Status as of 1st of January 2012), SR 830.1, ATSG.

Casillas, A., et al., "The Border of Reproductive Control: Undocumented Immigration as a Risk Factor for Unintended Pregnancy in Switzerland", *Journal of Immigrant Minority Health* 17 (2015), pp. 527–34, http://doi.org/10.1007/s10903-013-9939-9

Casino, G., "Spanish Health Cuts Could Create 'Humanitarian Problem'", *The Lancet* 379 (May 2012), p. 1777, https://doi.org/10.1016/s0140-6736(12)60745-4

Castaneda, H., "Illegality as Risk Factor: A Survey of Unauthorized Migrant Patients in a Berlin Clinic", *Social Science & Medicine* 68 (2009), pp. 1552–60, http://doi.org/10.1016/j.socscimed.2009.01.024

Castaneda, H., et al., "Immigration as a Social Determinant of Health", *Annual Review of Public Health* 36 (2015), pp. 375–92, http://doi.org/10.1146/annurev-publhealth-032013-182419

Cerri, C., et al., «Psychotropic Drugs Prescription in Undocumented Migrants and Indigent Natives in Italy», *International Clinical Psychopharmacy* 32.2 (2017), pp. 294–97, http://doi.org/10.1097/YIC.0000000000000184

Chiementi, M., et al., *La Répression du Travail Clandestin à Genève. Application des Sanctions et Conséquences pour les Personnes Concernées. Rapport de Recherche 27 du Forum Suisse pour l'Etude des Migrations et de la Population*, Neuchâtel, SFM/FSM 2003.

Cimas, M., et al., "Healthcare Coverage for Undocumented Migrants in Spain: Regional Differences after Royal Decree Law 16/2012", *Health Policy* 120 (2016), pp. 384–95, http://doi.org/10.1016/j.healthpol.2016.02.005

Clandestino Project, *Size and Development of Irregular Migration to the EU. Counting the Uncountable* (irregular-migration.net 2009), http://irregular-migration.net/typo3_upload/groups/31/4.Background_Information/4.2.Policy_Briefs_EN/ComparativePolicyBrief_SizeOfIrregularMigration_Clandestino_Nov09_2.pdf

Corbin, J. and A. Srauss, "Grounded Theory Research: Procedures, Canons and Evaluative Criteria", *Zeitschrift für Soziologie* 19.6 (1990), pp. 418–27.

Dauvin, M., et al., "Health Care for Irregular Migrants: Pragmatism Across Europe", *BMC Research Notes* 5.99 (2012), http://doi.org/10.1186/1756-0500-5-99

De Pietro, C., et al., «Switzerland. Health System Review", *Health Systems in Transition* 17.4 (2015), http://www.euro.who.int/__data/assets/pdf_file/0010/293689/Switzerland-HiT.pdf

Der Schweizerische Bundesrat: Vorläufige Aufnahme und Schutzbedürftigkeit: Analyse und Handlungsoptionen. Bericht in Erfüllung der Postulate 11.3954; 13.3844; 14.3008, Bern, 2016, https://www.sem.admin.ch/dam/data/sem/aktuell/news/2016/2016-10-14/ber-va-d.pdf

Devillanova, Carlo, "Social Networks, Information and Health Care Utilization: Evidence from Undocumented Immigrants in Milan", *Journal of Health Economics* 27 (2008), pp. 265–86. http://doi.org/10.1016/j.jhealeco.2007.08.006

De Vito, E., et al., "Are Undocumented Migrants' Entitlements and Barriers to Healthcare a Public Health Challenge for the European Union?", *Public Health Review* 37.13 (2016), http://doi.org/10.1186/s40985-016-0026-3

Dixon-Woods, M., et al., "Conducting a Critical Interpretive Synthesis of the Literature on Access to Healthcare by Vulnerable Groups", *BMC Medical Research Methodology* 6.35 (2006), http://doi:10.1186/1471-2288-6-35

Domnich, A., et al., "The 'Healthy Immigrant' Effect: Does it Exist in Europe Today?", *Italian Journal of Public Health* 9.3 (2012), p. e7532, http://doi.org/10.2427/7532

Efionayi-Mäder, D., et al., *Visage des Sans-Papiers en Suisse. Evolution 2000–2010*, Bern, Commission Fédérale pour les Questions de Migration CFM 2010, https://www.ekm.admin.ch/dam/data/ekm/dokumentation/materialien/mat_sanspap_f.pdf

Falla, A. M., et al., "Limited Access to Hepatitis B/C Treatment Among Vulnerable Risk Populations: An Expert Survey in Six European Countries", *European Journal of Public Health* 27.2 (2016), pp. 302–06, http://doi.org/10.1093/eurpub/ckw100

Federal Constitution of the Swiss Confederation of 18 April 1999 (Status as of 1 January 2016), SR 101, BV, https://www.admin.ch/opc/en/classified-compilation/19995395/index.html

Fiorini, G., et al., "The Burden of Chronic Noncommunicable Diseases in Undocumented Migrants: A 1-Year Survey of Drugs Dispensation by a Non-Governmental Organization in Italy", *Public Health* 141 (2016), pp. 26–31, http://doi.org/10.1016/j.puhe.2016.08.009

Fleischmann, Y., "Migration as a Social Determinant of Health for Irregular Migrants: Israel as a Case Study", *Social Science & Medicine* 147 (2015), pp. 89–97.

Frontex, Annual Risk Analysis 2015, Warsaw 2015, https://data.europa.eu/euodp/en/data/dataset/ara-2015

Frontex, Annual Risk Analysis 2016, Warsaw 2016, https://frontex.europa.eu/assets/Publications/Risk_Analysis/Annula_Risk_Analysis_2016.pdf

Glaser, B. and A. Strauss, *The Discovery of Grounded Theory. Strategies for Qualitative Research*, New Brunswick, Aldine Transaction 2006 [1967].

Gushulak, B., "Healthier on Arrival? Further Insight into the 'Healthy Migrant Effect'", *Canadian Medical Association Journal* 176.10 (2007), pp. 1439–40, http://doi.org/10.1503/cmaj.070395

Hacker, K., et al., "Barriers to Health Care for Undocumented Immigrants", *Risk Management and Healthcare Policy* 8 (2015), pp. 175–83, https://doi.org/10.2147/RMHP.S70173

Haenssgen, M. and A. Proochista, "Healthcare Access: A Sequence-Sensitive Approach", *SSM Population Health* 3 (2017), pp. 37–47, https://doi.org/10.1016/j.ssmph.2016.11.008

Heeren, M., et al., "Psychopathology and Resident Status — Comparing Asylum Seekers, Refugees, Illegal Migrants, and Residents", *Comprehensive Psychiatry* 55 (2014), pp. 818–25, https://doi.org/10.1016/j.comppsych.2014.02.003

Huschke, S., "Fragile Fabric: Illegality Knowledge, Social Capital and Health-Seeking of Undocumented Latin American Migrants in Berlin", *Journal of Ethnic and Migration Studies* 40.12 (2014), pp. 2010–29, https://doi.org/10.108 0/1369183X.2014.907740

Ikram, U. Z., et al., "Association between Immigration Policies and Immigrants' Mortality: An Explorative Study Across Three European Countries", *PLoS One* 10.6 (2015), http://doi.org/10.1371/journal.pone.0129916

IOM, *World Migration Report 2010*, Geneva, International Organization for Migration 2010, https://publications.iom.int/system/files/pdf/wmr_2010_english.pdf

Jandl, Michael, "The Estimation of Illegal Migration in Europe", *Migration Studies* 41.153 (2004), pp. 141–55.

Karlsen, M., "Migration Control and Childrens' Access to Health Care", in F. Thomas (ed.), *Handbook of Migration and Health*, Cheltenham, Edward Elgar Publishing 2016, pp. 134–57.

Kotsioni, I., "Irregular Migration and Health Challenges", in A. Triandafyllidou (ed.), *The Routledge Handbook of Immigration and Refugee Studies*, London and New York, Routledge 2016, pp. 371–77.

Kuehne, A., et al., "Subjective Health of Undocumented Migrants in Germany", *BMC Public Health* 15 (2015), pp. 916, http://doi.org/10.1186/s12889-015-2268-2

Lampart, D., et al., *Höhere Prämienverbilligungen gegen die Krankenkassen-Prämienlast*. Dossier No. 108, Schweizerischer Gewerkschaftsbund 2015.

Lampart, D., et al., *SGB-Verteilungsbericht 2016. Eine Analyse der Lohn- Einkommens- und Vermögensverteilung in der Schweiz*. Dossier No. 117, Schweizerischer Gewerkschaftsbund 2016.

Laranché, S., "Intangible Obstacles: Health Implications of Stigmatization, Structural Violence and Fear Among Undocumented Migrants in France", *Social Science & Medicine* 74 (2012), pp. 858–63, http://doi.org/10.1016/j.socscimed.2011.08.016

Legido-Quigley, H., et al., "Will Austerity Cuts Dismantle the Spanish Healthcare System?", *British Medical Journal*, 2013, http://doi.org/10.1136/bmj.f2363

Lvesque, J., et al., "Patient-Centred Access to Health Care: Conceptualising Access at the Interface of Health Systems and Populations", *International Journal for Equity in Health* 12.18 (2013), http://doi.org/10.1186/1475-9276-12-18

Lewis, G., "Health as an Elusive Concept" in H. Macbeth, and P. Shetty (eds.), *Health and Ethnicity*, London, Taylor & Francis, 2001.

Longchamp, C., *Sans Papiers in der Schweiz: Arbeitsmarkt, nicht Asylpolitik ist Entscheidend. Schlussbericht im Auftrag des Bundesamtes für Migration*, Bern, gfs 2005.

Luhmann, Niklas, *Die Gesellschaft der Gesellschaft*, Frankfurt a. M., Suhrkamp 1997.

Luhmann, Niklas, *Soziale Systeme. Grundriss einer Allgemeinen Theorie*, Frankfurt a. M., Suhrkamp 1991.

Marks-Sultan, G., et al., "The Legal and Ethical Aspects of the Right to Health of Migrants in Switzerland", *Public Health Review* 37.15 (2016), http://doi.org/10.1186/s40985-016-0027-2

Martinez, O., et al., "Evaluating the Impact of Immigration Policies on Health Status Among Undocumented Migrants", *Journal of Immigrant Minority Health* 17 (2015), pp. 947–70, http://doi.org/10.1007/s10903-013-9968-4

Morlok, M., et al., *Sans Papiers in der Schweiz 2015*, Schlussbericht zu Handen des Staatssekretariats für Migration (SEM), Basel 2015. https://www.sem.admin.ch/dam/data/sem/internationales/illegale-migration/sans_papiers/ber-sanspapiers-2015-d.pdf

Nassehi, A. and G. Nollmann, "Organisationssoziologische Ergänzungen der Inklusions-/Exklusionstheorie", *Soziale Systeme* 3.2 (1997), pp. 393–411.

Piccoli, L., *Left Out by the State, Taken in by the Region? Explaining the Regional Variation of Healthcare Rights for Undocumented Migrants in Italy, Spain and Switzerland*, Working Paper No. 10, Neuchâtel: NCCR on the move 2016, http://doc.rero.ch/record/288843

PICUM (Platform for International Cooperation on Undocumented Immigrants), *Access to Healthcare for Undocumented Migrants in Europe*, Brussels 2007, http://www.migration4development.org/sites/m4d.emakina-eu.net/files/paper_michelle_levoy.pdf

Piguet, E., *L'Immigration en Suisse*, Lausanne, Presses Polytechniques et Universitaires 2013.

Poduval, S., et al., "Experiences among Undocumented Migrants Accessing Primary Care in the United Kingdom", *International Journal of Health Services* 45.2 (2015), pp. 320–33, http://doi.org/10.1177/0020731414568511

Pool, R. and W. Geissler, *Medical Anthropology*, Berkshire, McGraw-Hill Education 2005.

Rechel, B., "Migration and Health in an Increasingly Diverse Europe", *The Lancet* 381 (2013), https://doi.org/10.1016/S0140-6736(12)62086-8

Roura, M., et al., "Carrying Ibuprofen in the Bag: Priority Health Concerns of Latin American Migrants in Spain — A Participatory Qualitative Study", *PLoS One* 10.8 (2015), http://doi.org/10.1371/journal.pone.0136315

Rossini, S. and V. Legrand-Germanier, *Le Système de Santé. Politique, Assurance, Médecine, Soins et Prévention*, Lausanne, Presses Polytechniques et Universitaires 2010.

Rüefli, C. and E. Huegli, *Krankenversicherung und Gesundheitsversorgung von Sans Papiers*, Bericht zur Beantwortung des Postulats Heim, Bern, Büro Vatter 2011.

Ruud, S. E., et al., "Use of Emergency Care Services by Immigrants — A Survey of Walk-in Patients Who Attended the Oslo Accident and Emergency Outpatient Clinic", *BMC Emergency Medicine* 15.25 (2015), http://doi.org/10.1186/s12873-015-0055-0

Sebo, P., et al., "Sexual and Reproductive Health Behaviours of Undocumented Migrants in Geneva", *Journal of Immigrant and Minority Health* 13 (2011), pp. 510–17, http://doi.org/10.1007/s10903-010-9367-z

SGK Kommission für Soziale Sicherheit und Gesundheit, *Für eine kohärente Gesetzgebung zu Sans-Papiers*, Motion No. 18.3005, 2018, https://www.parlament.ch/de/ratsbetrieb/suche-curia-vista/geschaeft?AffairId=20183005

Sigona, N. and V. Hughes, *No Way Out, No Way In: Irregular Children and Families in the UK*, Research Report, Oxford, ESRC Centre on Migration, Policy and Society, University of Oxford, 2012, https://www.compas.ox.ac.uk/media/PR-2012-Undocumented_Migrant_Children.pdf

Sozialversicherungsanstalt des Kantons Zürich, *Merkblatt. Höhe der Jährlichen Prämienverbilligung 2017*, https://www.svazurich.ch/pdf/IPV2017_Hoehe.pdf

Staatssekretariat für Migration: Asylstatistik 2016, Bern 2017, https://www.sem.admin.ch/sem/de/home/publiservice/statistik/asylstatistik/archiv/2016.html

Stichweh, R., *Inklusion und Exklusion in der Weltgesellschaft — Am Beispiel der Schule und des Erziehungssystems*, 2007, https://www.fiw.uni-bonn.de/demokratieforschung/personen/stichweh/pdfs/97_stw_inklusion-und-exklusion-in-der-weltgesellschaft-schule-und-erziehungssystem.pdf

Stichweh, R., *Inklusion und Exklusion. Studien zur Gesellschaftstheorie*, Bielefeld, Transcript 2005.

Strassmayr, C., et al., "Mental Health Care for Irregular Migrants in Europe: Barriers and How They Are Overcome", *BMC Public Health* 12 (2012), pp. 367, https://doi.org/10.1186/1471-2458-12-367

Swiss Civil Code of 10 December 1907 (Status as of 1 January 2017), SR 210, ZGB, https://www.admin.ch/opc/en/classified-compilation/19070042/index.html

UK Parliament, Health and Social Care Committee, Memorandum of Understanding on Data-sharing Inquiry (16 January 2018), https://www.parliament.uk/business/committees/committees-a-z/commons-select/health-committee/inquiries/parliament-2017/mou-data-sharing-nhs-digital-home-office-inquiry-17-19/

Valli, M., *Les Migrants sans Permis de Séjour à Lausanne. Rapport Rédigé à la Demande de la Municipalité de Lausanne*, 2003, http://www.sans-papiers.ch/fileadmin/redaktion/Hintergrund/5FRStudie_Sans-P._in_Lausanne_2003.pdf

Vazquez, M. L., et al., "Are Migrants Health Policies Aimed at Improving Access to Quality Healthcare? An Analysis of Spanish Policies", *Health Policy* 113 (2013), pp. 236–46, https://doi.org/10.1016/j.healthpol.2013.06.007

Verein SansPapiersCare, *Gesundheitsversorgung von Sans Papiers in Acht Westeuropäischen Staaten*, Zürich, 2016.

Verordnung über die Krankenversicherung vom 27. Juni 1995 (Status as of 1 March 2017), SR 832.102, KVV, https://www.admin.ch/opc/de/classified-compilation/19950219/index.html

Vogel, D., et al., "The Size of Irregular Migrant Population in the European Union — Counting the Uncountable?", *International Migration* 49.5 (2011), pp. 78–96, http://doi.org/10.1111/j.1468-2435.2011.00700.x

Weidtmann, J., *Paradoxien in der Regulierung von Migration. Schwierigkeiten von Sans-Papiers in der Schweiz bei der Wahrnehmung des Rechts auf Krankenversicherung*, Bachelor thesis, Institut für Sozialanthropologie Universität Bern, 2015, http://sanspapiersbern.ch/wp-content/uploads/2015/11/Bachelorarbeit_Johanna-Weidtmann-.pdf

Weiss, R., *Confronting Cultural Challenges for Migrant Health Care in Switzerland*, Independent Study Project (ISP) Collection (Spring 2015), http://digitalcollections.sit.edu/cgi/viewcontent.cgi?article=3136&context=isp_collection

Wolff, H. and M. Epiney, "Undocumented Migrants Lack Access to Pregnancy Care and Prevention", *BMC Public Health* 8.93 (2008), http://doi.org/10.1186/1471-2458-8-93

Woodward, A., et al., "Health and Access to Care for Undocumented Migrants Living in the European Union", *Health Policy and Planning*, 2013, pp. 1–13, http://doi.org/10.1093/heapol/czt061

Wysmüller, C. and D. Efionayi-Mäder, *Undocumented Migrants' Needs and Strategies to Access Health Care in Switzerland & Practices of Health Care Provision*, Wien, International Center for Migration Policy Development, 2011.

Zimmermann, C., et al., "Migration and Health: A Framework for 21st Century Policy Making", *PLoS Medicine* 8.5 (2011), http://doi.org/10.1371/journal.pmed.1001034

This book need not end here…

At Open Book Publishers, we are changing the nature of the traditional academic book. The title you have just read will not be left on a library shelf, but will be accessed online by hundreds of readers each month across the globe. OBP publishes only the best academic work: each title passes through a rigorous peer-review process. We make all our books free to read online so that students, researchers and members of the public who can't afford a printed edition will have access to the same ideas.

This book and additional content is available at:

https://www.openbookpublishers.com/product/748

Customize

Personalize your copy of this book or design new books using OBP and third-party material. Take chapters or whole books from our published list and make a special edition, a new anthology or an illuminating coursepack. Each customized edition will be produced as a paperback and a downloadable PDF. Find out more at:

https://www.openbookpublishers.com/section/59/1

Donate

If you enjoyed this book, and feel that research like this should be available to all readers, regardless of their income, please think about donating to us. We do not operate for profit and all donations, as with all other revenue we generate, will be used to finance new Open Access publications.

https://www.openbookpublishers.com/section/13/1/support-us

[f] Like Open Book Publishers

[twitter] Follow @OpenBookPublish

BLOG Read more at the OBP Blog

You may also be interested in:

Intellectual Property and Public Health
in the Developing World

By Monirul Azam

https://www.openbookpublishers.com/product/476

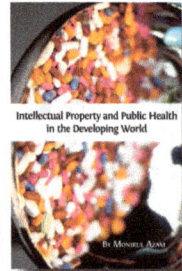

World of Walls
The Structure, Roles and Effectiveness
of Separation Barriers

By Said Saddiki

https://www.openbookpublishers.com/product/635

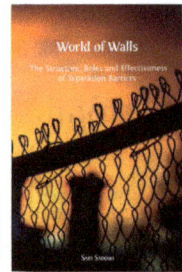

Wellbeing, Freedom and Social Justice
The Capability Approach Re-Examined

By Ingrid Robeyns

https://www.openbookpublishers.com/product/682

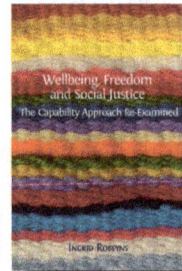

The Universal Declaration of Human Rights
in the 21st Century
A living document in a changing world

Edited by Gordon Brown

https://www.openbookpublishers.com/product/467

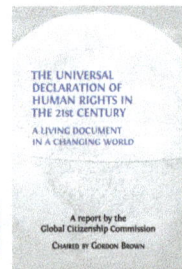

www.ingramcontent.com/pod-product-compliance
Lightning Source LLC
Chambersburg PA
CBHW071749270326
41928CB00013B/2852